Health in a Bottle

SEARCHING FOR THE DRUGS THAT HELP

Health in a Bottle

SEARCHING FOR THE DRUGS THAT HELP

L. EARLE ARNOW, PhD, MD

Senior Scientific Consultant
Warner-Lambert Research Institute
Morris Plains, New Jersey

Philadelphia & Toronto

J. B. LIPPINCOTT COMPANY

1970

Dedicated to

DR. WILLIAM A. FEIRER

*who first brought me into the pharmaceutical industrial
research community in 1942, and who has been a
warm friend and a wise mentor ever since*

ACKNOWLEDGMENT

Many people have given me a helping hand during the writing of this book and I am grateful to all of them. I owe special thanks to Dr. Karl Bambach, for many years a senior member of the staff of the Pharmaceutical Manufacturers Association. He has read each chapter as it was written, and his constructive criticisms have increased the readability and accuracy of these chapters.

We are also grateful to a number of pharmaceutical companies for sending us pictures and permitting their use in *Health in a Bottle:* Bristol Laboratories, Hoffmann-La Roche Laboratories, Inc., Merck Sharp & Dohme, Chas. Pfizer & Co., Inc., Smith Kline & French Laboratories, and the Warner-Lambert Research Institute. Each picture or group of pictures is acknowledged by an obvious abbreviation at the end of the legend for it.

Contents

CHAPTER 1

Overture

The Search for New Drugs, *Ethical* and
Proprietary, The Cost, The Searchers,
The Benefits

THE SEARCH FOR NEW DRUGS in the laboratories of the United
States pharmaceutical industry is, to the scientists who engage
in it, exciting, interesting, and, all too often, frustrating. This
research is expensive; it cannot be evaluated with the tools
ordinarily used to evaluate business endeavors; and yet it is
essential for economic survival. To the physician and his patients, it is the major source for new (and, occasionally,
spectacular) therapeutic agents. In the period from 1940
through 1966, more than 800 major new drugs were made
available to the American physician and his patients. Approximately two thirds of these originated in the laboratories of the
American pharmaceutical industry. None came from countries
behind the Iron Curtain.

The odds for success in the search for new drugs are almost
unbelievably small. A survey conducted in 1967 indicated that
the American pharmaceutical industry subjects approximately
175,000 substances to biologic evaluation each year. This number may be higher today, but that is not certain. More scientists are engaged in pharmaceutical research and development
today, but the man-hours required for the discovery and development of a new drug also have increased markedly. To be
conservative, I shall use the figure 175,000 in making the following estimate. Each time a substance is evaluated biologically, of course, one hopes that this first biologic study will

9

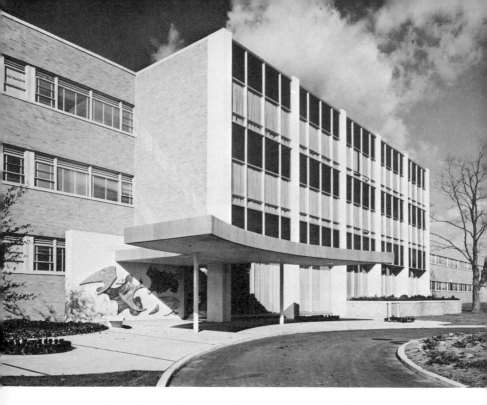

The Warner-Lambert Research Institute, Morris Plains, New Jersey

be the initial step in the gestation and birth of a new drug. Alas! Judging from recent past experience, some 20 of these 175,000 substances will make the grade. The odds, then, are a frustrating one to 8,750. In the special case of new synthetic chemicals, the odds are a little more favorable, but not much more. My own estimate is that one in 60 new chemicals submitted for biologic testing shows enough promise to justify an appreciable amount of additional laboratory investigation. Probably not more than one in 240 is found to be sufficiently potent yet sufficiently low in toxicity to justify testing it in human subjects. One of every 10 compounds subjected to clinical trial in humans may become a new drug. The odds, then, are 1 in 2,400. When all types of samples submitted to biologic evaluation are considered (including, as one example, broths in which microorganisms have been grown in an antibiotic screening program), the odds decrease to about 1 in 8,750.

Why are these odds so low? One important reason is that scientists do not know enough about the relationship between chemical structure and biologic activity to be able to predict the biologic properties of a *completely new chemical compound*. These last words I italicize because often the activity of a new compound, whose chemical structure differs only slightly from that of an established drug, can be predicted; it will be qualitatively the same as that of the drug in many cases. If the chemist begins his synthetic program with such a compound—in other words, if he is planning to modify the structure of a known drug he can use his chemical expertise to make new compounds that may have advantages compared to the parent drug. For example, the research may lead to a drug with greater clinical activity, lesser toxicity, better absorption from the gastrointestinal tract, greater physical stability, or lower cost to the patient.

A difficulty even more serious is that we simply do not have enough laboratory tests in animals that are predictive of clinical utility for humans. Most of the animals used in biologic studies are *healthy*. Indeed, most of the diseases that afflict man cannot be reproduced in animals. One good reason for this is our lack of knowledge about the fundamental causes of such diseases as cancer, heart disease, mental disease, diabetes mellitus, peptic ulcer, allergy, and most others. In the laboratory we use models that we hope will be useful in leading us to new drugs that will be active in the clinic. For example, cortisone and some other compounds chemically related to it have been found to have activity in relieving many of the signs and symptoms of rheumatoid arthritis. Yet these same compounds have activity in laboratory tests that bear only superficial resemblance to arthritis in the human. One of the first successful tests consisted in placing a small piece of cotton under the skin of a rat. After a week or longer, it was removed and weighed. During its stay in the animal it gained weight, partly because it absorbed fluid and partly because the animal's tissue reacted to this foreign body by depositing a tissue barrier around it. Corticoids (drugs having the biologic and clinical activity of cortisone), if given to the animal during this experiment, had the ability to decrease this gain in weight. It was assumed in some laboratories that new compounds active in this animal test would be active also in clinical arthritis. This was true for new drugs closely related chemically to cortisone, but some of the newer drugs now used in the management of arthritis are not related chemically to cortisone and show very little activity in the cotton pellet test. The most common cause of failure during the laboratory studies of a potential new therapeutic agent is toxicity; the most common cause of failure in the clinic is lack of effectiveness.

Among the modern drugs, the most useful are those that are effective in the treatment of infectious diseases—the sulfonamides and the antibiotics are prime examples. Fortunately, it is possible often to reproduce the infectious human disease in the animal. Ordinarily, the experimental conditions are such that the infected animals will die if they are not protected by the administration of an effective agent. Weaker agents that might be useful in the therapy of mild infections in humans undoubtedly have been overlooked, because they are not effective in combating the overwhelming infections used in the laboratory screen. On the negative side, also, is the distressing fact that none of the available antiinfective drugs is active against systemic infections caused by viruses. A number of viral infections can be reproduced in animals, but the blind screening of thousands of chemicals and potential antibiotic-containing broths has not yielded a clinically effective agent.

For a time, particularly during the second 25 years of this century, the isolation and synthesis of vitamins was a prime effort of the young pharmaceutical research community. Some of the diseases caused by a lack of vitamins in the diet were recognized centuries before the first vitamin was isolated. Scurvy, caused by a deficiency of ascorbic acid (vitamin C) was a prevalent disease in Europe as early as 1400 AD. Beri-beri, caused by a deficiency of thiamine (vitamin B_1), has been common in the Far East since the time its inhabitants began to use polished rice as a major item of the diet. The discarded hulls contained the precious vitamin. Rickets, caused by a double deficiency of phosphate and vitamin D, has been known for at least 350 years.

Following the birth and development of the new science of nutrition in the early part of this century, it became possible to search for vitamins in the laboratory. The procedure was to feed diets prepared by mixing relatively pure components to laboratory animals, most commonly the rat. As the vitamins already found became available, they, or concentrates of them, were added to the diet, as were the necessary minerals and water. If the animals failed to grow at a normal rate, or exhibited other signs of abnormality, it was assumed that one or more unknown vitamins were missing from the diet. Other animals were fed the original diet, supplemented by different natural foods, until a good source of the unknown vitamin was found. After a time, it was discovered that certain microorganisms would not grow unless the necessary vitamins were added to the culture medium. Since bacteria grow much faster than animals, their use considerably shortened the time required for experiment. It was found also that many microorganisms *syn-*

thesized vitamins during their growth. Broths containing these vitamins of microbial origin proved to be convenient sources that the chemists could use in isolating the new vitamins. The availability of microbial sources and rapid microbial screening tests made it possible for chemists to isolate, purify, identify, and synthesize the 20 or so recognized vitamins within a relatively short span of years. However, no new vitamin required by the human has been found for a number of years, and the search for such agents no longer is an interesting, or probably an important, endeavor.

Another type of natural product is the hormone. One of them, epinephrine (adrenaline, first isolated from the medulla, or core, of the adrenal gland) was prepared in pure form in 1901. Desiccated (dried) thyroid gland and extracts of this gland have been available to the physician for many years. Insulin, the pancreatic hormone used in the management of diabetes mellitus, was marketed in the early 1920s. A number of hormones are known to be made by the anterior pituitary gland, but only two of them are marketed as drugs. One of them is adrenocorticotropic hormone (ACTH, or corticotropin); it stimulates the patient's own adrenal cortex (outer part of the gland) to secrete cortisone-like hormones. The other, thyrotropin (thyroid-stimulating hormone, TSH) causes the thyroid gland to secrete its hormone. The pituitary hormones, as well as the hypothalamic hormones (which regulate the discharge of the hormones of the pituitary gland into the blood stream), are extremely complex chemically and cannot practicably be prepared synthetically. (ACTH has been made synthetically in the laboratory.) Moreover, disturbing evidence indicates that some of these hormones of animal origin may not be active in the human. The posterior pituitary gland makes two hormones. They have been synthesized, and one of them—oxytocin—is used in obstetrics.

Since late in 1944, when Dr. Lewis H. Sarett of the Merck Research Laboratories synthesized the hormone, cortisone, a number of corticoids (compounds related chemically to cortisone and having its clinical activity) have been introduced as drugs. The male and female sex hormones, related chemically to cortisone but having very different biologic properties, were isolated and synthesized in the 1930s. These substances have been used as therapeutic agents for many years, but only in the recent past were combinations of substances possessing the biologic activities of the female sex hormones found to be capable of preventing conception in the human. Other known hormones occur in the parathyroid glands and in the gastrointestinal tract; they have very limited usefulness as therapeutic agents at the present time. Two other hormones—one made in the thyroid and one made in the thymus—are known, but their possible utility cannot be assessed until they have been studied intensively in the clinic. The new hormone from the thyroid (thyrocalcitonin) has been synthesized, the hormone from the thymus (thymosin) has been partially purified.

Enzymes are substances that make it possible for most of the essential chemical reactions that take place in the body to occur. For example, they are essential for the digestion of food. Some of them are used as drugs, but, in general, their field of usefulness is small.

Antibiotics are substances of natural origin, since they are made by microorganisms. It is true that some of them, especially penicillin, have been modified in a useful way by the chemist. It is becoming increasingly more difficult, however, to find new ones of value in medicine. More than 1,000 antibiotics have been discovered and studied; less than 30 are used as drugs.

Obviously, one way to search for new drugs is to discover evidence for the existence of naturally occurring substances of potential medicinal value and to isolate, characterize, and study them. Of course this field of research is under investigation in many research centers, most of them outside the pharmaceutical industry. This is a difficult method of attack and the odds of success are extremely small. Another approach, most common in the pharmaceutical industry, is to make new synthetic chemicals and to study them in biologic systems. An important limiting factor here is the biologic knowledge that makes it possible to devise meaningful tests of activity. In other words, until new biologic test systems can be set up, the new chemicals can be tested only in systems known to be predictive of activities possessed by already known drugs. For this reason, the search for such systems is an important part of the research effort in the pharmaceutical industry.

The research we have been discussing is related to *ethical* drugs. The word *ethical* has a special meaning in the vocabulary of the pharmaceutical industry. An ethical drug is one that is advertised or promoted only to members of the health professions—for example, to physicians, pharmacists, dentists, veterinarians, nurses. In most cases, ethical drugs are sold only on prescription, but there are some exceptions to this: for example, most antacids and vitamin formulations. *Proprietary* drugs, on the other hand, are advertised and promoted to the public—via television, radio, newspapers, popular magazines, mailing of samples to the home, and so on. Of course it would be entirely incorrect, even in the jargon of the pharmaceutical industry, to characterize these drugs as unethical. To make things even more confusing, the adjective *proprietary* has another meaning. The proprietary name of a drug is the brand name or trademark used by a specific manufacturer. The common or generic name of a drug is used by all companies that sell it, but each may, if it chooses, identify the product by a proprietary name that cannot legally be used by others.

Obviously, proprietary drugs are recognized as safe enough to be used without medical supervision. In most cases, this limits the proprietary drug field to medicinal agents that have been used for many years and by millions of people, so that safety has been established. For this reason, almost every new drug must be introduced to the market as an "ethical" product.

Ethical drugs can be placed into two categories. An *entity* means a drug that is a single chemical substance or a single biologic product (such as measles vaccine). The other type of product consists of a mixture of entities, and it is referred to as a *combination drug*. Either type may be prepared in different dosage forms—for examples, as tablets, syrups, solutions for injection, and so on. Sometimes, in discussing the new products that are marketed within a calendar year, the phrase *new entities* is used. This simply means the entities that have appeared on the market for the first time. Entities from previous years that may appear in new dosage forms are excluded.

Because it is impossible to predict exactly, even within years, when a new drug will be discovered, and because its economic importance usually cannot be evaluated exactly prior to marketing, pharmaceutical industrial research cannot be evaluated by the economic tools ordinarily used by business management. In 1965, the pharmaceutical industry spent one million dollars a day—including Saturdays, Sundays, and holidays—in ethical pharmaceutical research and development. The total figure reported for the year was $365.1 million. A small amount of this money ($13.7 million) was furnished by the Government, and another small amount ($22.7 million) was used in the search for veterinary drugs. The amount of Industry money spent in drugs for humans, then, was $328.7 million in 1965. (The amount estimated for 1968 was $521 million—almost $2 million for every working day.)

If none of this money had been spent—that is, if no ethical

research and development in the human field had been carried out in the Industry—the companies could have retained approximately $170.9 million. The remainder would have been lost as income tax. (A tax rate of 48 percent has been assumed in making this calculation.) The average net profit after taxes for the Industry in 1965 was 10.7 percent of net sales. In order to recoup the $170.9 million in income after taxes, then—that is, as income that could be used for dividends and for business expenditures requiring cash—future sales amounting to $1.6 billion would have to be generated. Now suppose that management expects to regain this money by the sale of significant new drugs, that is, by the sale of new entities. There were 23 of these marketed in 1965. The estimated sales, at manufacturer's level, generated by these new entities in the first full year of marketing, 1966, was $77 million. Even if this rate of sales continued indefinitely, almost 21 years would be required to generate $1.6 billion of sales. Obviously, that is absurd. For one thing, approximately one third of these sales was accounted for by one product and 85 percent of the sales were from half of them. Moreover, almost 70 percent of the ethical drugs sold in 1965 did not even exist in 1955.

Perhaps it is unwise to pursue this type of computation too far—or to draw any sweeping conclusions from it, except to decide that it is difficult to evaluate the productivity of a research group in terms of new entities discovered and marketed. Actually the new entities marketed in 1965 were financed almost entirely by funds expended in previous years, since a number of years are necessary for the development of a new entity even after it is discovered in the laboratory. Moreover, in 1965 more than 100 ethical products were marketed. Some of these were old entities in new dosage forms; others were combination dosage forms. The total ethical sales of $4.2 billion for 1965, then, came from drugs marketed in previous years, from newly marketed ethical products that were not new entities, and from new entities.

Some combination dosage forms are extremely useful to the physician and to his patient, and these can be very important economically to the firm that supplies them. An obvious example is the various contraceptive tablets now on the market. They are combinations of two types of female sex hormone or, more exactly, of compounds that have the biologic activities of these hormones.

Many of the ethical products are marketed by small firms and do not contribute significantly to total sales for the Industry. Most of the ethical sales are accounted for by about half of the 140 members of the Pharmaceutical Manufacturers Association. Almost two thirds of the United States market results from the activities of the 13 firms that had individual global sales exceeding $100 million in 1965 and these same companies accounted for about two thirds of the research and development expenditures.

The small firms simply cannot afford to search for new entities. It is estimated that each new drug discovered during the past decade has cost on the average $5 million, and this cost increases each year. If every member of the research community having a bachelor's degree or equivalent is regarded as a scientist, then $36,000 annually is required to keep one scientist on the job. Fifty five percent of the total personnel of the pharmaceutical research group has a professional degree; one-sixth of these professional people are women. Approximately 19,400 scientists and supporting technicians were engaged in research and development activities in the Industry in 1967.

The sales of ethical drugs almost doubled between 1951 and 1965. During this same period, research and development expenditures increased six times. During the last five years of the period, however, the rates of increase were not so far apart;

sales increased about 43 percent and research and development expenses about 47 percent. In 1965 funds supplied for R&D were 73 percent of the net profit after taxes. In past years, this figure has ranged from about 47 percent in 1950 to a high of 89 percent in 1952. For 1965, 73 percent is close to that for 1958 (76 percent). In 1963 R&D, financed by both federal and company funds for *all* US companies engaged in R&D, was 68 percent of net profit. If only company-financed R&D is considered (the fairest method of making a comparison with the ethical pharmaceutical industry), the figure falls to 29.5 percent.

R&D in the pharmaceutical industry differs from that in other industries in several interesting ways. In a typical chemical firm almost all of the professional staff are chemists or chemical engineers. The professional staff of a medium or large pharmaceutical group, by way of contrast, consists of a highly diverse group of specialists, including organic chemists, analytical chemists, physical chemists, chemical engineers, biochemists, physiologists, pharmacologists, bacteriologists, virologists, immunologists, toxicologists, pathologists, pharmacists, veterinarians, and physicians. Some groups have even more specialists: for example, parasitologists, enzymologists, dentists, nutritionists, and mycologists. In addition to the scientific staff, a large group of supporting personnel is required. It includes specialists in research management and administration, statistics, electronics, program planning, personnel, accounting, storage and retrieval of research data, library science, maintenance engineering, photography, medical and scientific writing and the graphic arts, shop working, and glass blowing. Of course, other industrial research organizations require some of these supporting skills also, although probably not all.

The ethical drug industry spends a higher percentage of

R&D funds for basic research than any other industry. The term "basic research" has been defined in many ways, but as applied here to industrial research organizations, it is defined as the planned search for new knowledge, whether or not the search has reference to a specific application. It contrasts with *a*) the application of existing knowledge to problems involved in the creation of a new product or process, including work required to evaluate possible uses, and *b*) application of existing knowledge to problems involved in the improvement of a present product or process.

Calculations made from figures compiled by the National Science Foundation for 1966 indicate that 15.1 percent of pharmaceutical R&D was basic research.* Figures for some other industries (including funds from both companies and government) were: industrial chemicals, 13.0 percent; petroleum refining and extraction, 7.5 percent; food and kindred products, 5.4 percent. The figures for other industries were lower still. The pharmaceutical industry has the highest ratio of company-financed R&D to net sales of any industry. According to the National Science Foundation, funds for all of industrial research in 1966 were 4.1 percent of net sales. This included money supplied by the Government. The figure for company-financed R&D was 1.9 percent in the same year. The figure for the pharmaceutical industry in 1966 for ethical R&D was 10.9 percent.

R&D financed by the company, to put this another way, amounted to $460 per employee for all industry conducting R&D in 1963. The figure reported by the National Science Foundation for the chemical and allied products industries (of which the pharmaceutical industry is one) was much higher, $1,030 per employee. The figure for the pharmaceutical

* A survey conducted by the Pharmaceutical Manufacturers Association in 1967 yielded a figure of 17.9 percent.

industry in 1965 was higher still, $1,500 per employee. Only 2.4 percent of pharmaceutical R&D is paid for with government money. According to the National Science Foundation, the figure for all industrial research in this country was 55 percent in 1965.

The pharmaceutical industry, for good reasons, is regulated by governmental agencies—the chief one, and certainly the most important to research and development, being the Food and Drug Administration (FDA), a part of the Department of Health, Education, and Welfare (HEW). The original bureau that later became the FDA was created in 1906, when the development and marketing of drugs was in a shameful state. Manufacturers could and *did* market any product with no quality control and with no clinical or laboratory study at all. Often these products were useless medically and almost always low in purity and quality. Even potent "prescription drugs," such as narcotics, were marketed over the counter without controls.

The law passed in 1906 established standards for drugs but was defective in that it did not control the development or marketing of drugs so long as these standards were met and the label on the package indicated accurately the names and quantities of active ingredients. In 1938, the defectiveness of the 1906 law was revealed, shockingly, when a liquid preparation containing sulfanilamide killed almost 100 people—it contained a toxic solvent that had not been tested adequately in animals or humans. A new law was passed providing that a new drug application (NDA) be submitted to the FDA prior to marketing. This was an attempt to insure that adequate toxicity studies had been made. In 1962, the present law was enacted—often referred to as the Kefauver-Harris Amendments—and it required that the FDA make a positive ruling that a new drug was sufficiently *safe* and *effective* prior to marketing. Actually this law might not have passed, at least in 1962, if it had not been for two events: one the disclosure of the horrid birth of several thousand defective babies abroad who had been exposed to a sedative, thalidomide, during pregnancy; the other, that when the bill was almost tabled in a subcommittee of the House, the Pharmaceutical Manufacturers Association (PMA) supported it. Thalidomide never was marketed in this country, but it was being tested clinically when the story broke, although the company sponsoring the studies had withdrawn its NDA. Strangely, perhaps, there was no question of the drug's effectiveness and very little established toxicity—except the dreadful effect on unborn babies. Moreover, there were no animal tests available in 1962 that would show this type of toxicity in animals for thalidomide. Nonetheless, it certainly triggered the passage of a law requiring evidence of safety and effectiveness of a new drug.

Much has been written about a running controversy between the FDA and the pharmaceutical industry regarding development and marketing of new drugs. Most of this comes about because the decision that a new drug is *safe* and *effective* is a judgment. No potent drug is entirely free of toxicity, and actually, some drugs used in the treatment of cancer are extremely toxic. No drug is completely efficacious, none will of itself cure cancer. It is natural, I think, for the FDA to prefer to err (if err it must) on the conservative side and to require a large (even vast, sometimes) amount of evidence before making its decision that the drug can be marketed. If a mistake is made, the agency will be subjected to intense criticism by the Government, the news media, and the people. On the other hand, the pharmaceutical industry is spending about $2 million each working day in the search for new drugs and understandably wishes to market a new drug as soon as, in the judgment of its own competent staffs of scientists and physicians, there is sufficient evidence. (The FDA is discussed more fully in Chapter 5. Some drugs, such as vaccines and blood plasma, are controlled by another group within HEW, The Division of Biologics Standards, discussed in Chapter 6.)

The most tangible benefits of the availability of new, potent drugs—many of them discovered in the laboratories of the US pharmaceutical industry—have been a lowered death rate; a decrease in the incidence, duration, and severity of illness; and, coupled with these, an increase in the average span of life in the United States. In 1930, just before the era of modern chemotherapy, life expectancy at birth was 59.7 years; in the years that followed, many lives were saved with the aid of the new drugs, and the life expectancy at birth rose to 70.2 years in 1965. Much of this gain resulted from the prevention of deaths due to infectious diseases in young people and infants, but there was some gain in the older age groups also. For example, a person 65 years old had a life expectancy of about 12 years in 1930; by 1965 this had increased to 15.2 years. The death rate (per 1,000 of population) for infants under one year of age was 69.0 in 1930; in 1965 it had dropped to 23.4. The rate decreased during the same period from 4.7 to 1.5 for young adults (25 to 34 years of age) and from 51.4 to 37.9 for the old (65 to 74 years of age). A decrease occurred even for persons aged 85 years or over—from 228.0 in 1930 to 202.2 in 1965.

According to the Metropolitan Life Insurance Company, when President and Mrs. Eisenhower were married, the chance that a man 26 years and a woman 19 years old both would live for 50 additional years was only one in 6; the odds now are one in 3. The Eisenhowers celebrated their golden (fiftieth year) wedding anniversary in 1966. Arthur D. Little, Inc., has estimated that 4,400,000 Americans were alive in 1960 who would have been dead if the death rates prevailing in 1935 had persisted. Americans between the ages of 15 and 64 who suffered from four diseases (tuberculosis, influenza, pneumonia, and syphilis) and were salvaged in 1960 alone were estimated to number 152,178. About two thirds of these (100,789) were employed; as a group they earned $411.9 million during the year. Another estimate indicated that in 1959 the net economic gain in this country due to reduction in days lost from work as a result of illness was $2.51 billion. An important social gain resulting from the increase in life expectancy is interesting. Termination of marriage by death now occurs at much older ages than before the age of modern therapeutic agents. As a result, fewer of today's children must pass through their dependency period without both parents.

As expected (in view of the increase in population in the older age group), the rate of admission to general hospitals has increased in recent years. This rate was 58.6 per 1,000 population in 1935; it had increased to 144.7 in 1964. At the same time, however, the average length of stay in the hospital fell from 15.0 days in 1935 to 9.2 days in 1964. The types of illness prevalent among hospitalized patients have also changed over the years. The number of cases of communicable disease has declined; this has been offset by a marked increase in the cases of chronic diseases, such as heart disease and cancer.

The price of prescription drugs tends to decline with the passage of time after introduction to the market. The United States Bureau of Labor Statistics annually prices 14 prescription drugs; 12 of these are among the 100 drugs prescribed most frequently. Using the years 1957-1959 as a base (100 percent), the consumer prices of all consumer commodities reached 115 percent in 1967; food prices were 114 percent. The selected prescription drug prices were 90 percent. The average prescription purchased in 1967 cost the patient $3.56. For the entire year, the average person spent less than $16 for prescription drugs. For persons over 65 years of age, the average cost was $41.40.

The distribution of the consumer's money spent for the average prescription in 1967 was approximately as follows:

DISTRIBUTION OF CONSUMER'S MONEY	RECEIPTS (cents)	EARNINGS & EXPENSES (cents)
Retailers received from consumers	356	
Retailer's prescription expenses		124
Retailer's earnings from prescriptions before taxes		36
Wholesalers received from retailers	196	
Wholesaler's prescription drug expenses		25
Wholesaler's earnings from prescription drugs before taxes		7
Manufacturers received from wholesalers	164	
Manufacturer's production expenses		54
Manufacturer's R&D expenses		18
Manufacturer's other expenses		53
Manufacturer's federal income tax expense		18
Manufacturer's earnings after taxes		21

Thus, of the $3.56 paid by the consumer for the average prescription in 1967, the manufacturer received a profit of 21¢ (5.9%) after taxes. Obviously elimination of, as an example, half of this profit would not help the consumer very much. If promotion and advertising costs of ethical drugs were lowered drastically, many physicians would not be well enough informed about new drugs to prescribe them intelligently. Seventeen percent of the workers, and 11 percent of the floor space in the manufacturing area, are occupied with quality control. Products often require as many as a hundred (sometimes, several hundred) analyses by quality control personnel between the raw material stage and shipment of the final product. If research and development expenses were eliminated or even decreased appreciably, the flow of new therapeutic agents—already slow enough—would decrease correspondingly.

CHAPTER 2

Gestation of a Synthetic Drug

From laboratory—to market or oblivion. By
way of biologic tests, basic research.
The scientists, the plans, the time

THE LIFE CYCLE of a synthetic drug usually begins in the laboratory of an organic chemist. He must start his synthetic program by choosing which one of three courses to pursue. One way is to choose to make compounds as closely related to a successful drug as he can. An obvious advantage is that the compounds he makes *may* have biologic activity qualitatively very similar to that of the known drug. The word *may* is italicized because similar biologic activity does not always occur; all too often, very slight changes in chemical structure abolish the desirable biologic activity. An obvious disadvantage exists if the established drug belongs to a competitive firm. The chemists of that firm, desiring a strong patent position and, of course, searching for the best possible compound in a series, probably have made a number of derivatives. Since patents do not become available for several years after an application is filed, our chemist may discover an interesting compound that cannot be marketed because it is covered by a patent.

The most obvious advantage of this line of attack, though, is that it offers an opportunity to discover a new drug in an area that is interesting therapeutically. One may hope that a new substance with advantages over the marketed drug may be found. The advantage might be, as examples, lower toxicity, better absorption and utilization, lower dosage, lower costs, or new properties that make it easier to produce stable, palatable dosage forms. Another possibility is that one of the new compounds, although related chemically to the old one, may have entirely different biologic effects. A number of important new drugs have been discovered as a result of attempts to improve old ones. For example, compounds useful in lowering the blood sugar of patients with diabetes mellitus came from studies of compounds related chemically to sulfanilamide.

Another method of attack is to develop a theoretical concept that suggests the type of compound to make. The chemist may postulate, for example, that the spatial relationships of the atoms in a molecule are responsible for its biologic activity. Entirely new structures having these spatial relationships can be made, and the hypothesis thus tested. A line of attack sometimes is suggested by something the chemist reads in the scientific literature. In 1940, T. Mann and D. Keilin in England published their observation that sulfanilamide is a powerful inhibitor of the enzyme carbonic anhydrase in the test tube. This observation really was the beginning of a long trail that led to the discovery of an important group of diuretic agents—the chlorothiazides.

A third possibility is to make entirely new kinds of compounds—chemical types that never have been made before. In this case, whether the compounds will have biologic activity, and if so what kind, is completely unknown. If such substances are subjected to a variety of biologic tests, interesting activity may be found. If so, perhaps a new type of drug may emerge. This approach led to the discovery of the widely used drug, Librium (Roche Laboratories' proprietary name for chlordiazepoxide hydrochloride).

So the chemist embarks on his synthetic program. As each new compound is made, he sends it to the analytical and physical chemistry laboratories, for two excellent reasons.

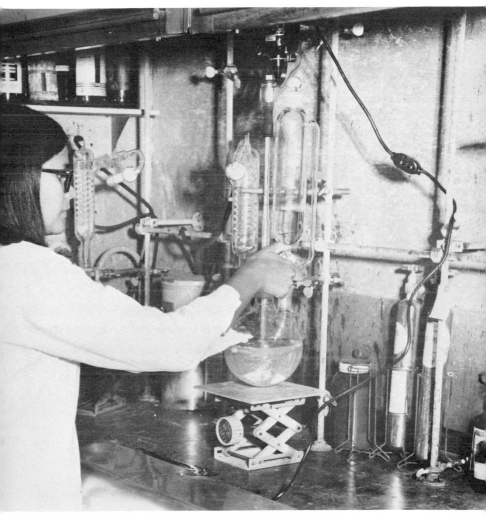

This chemist is making a new chemical compound that she hopes will become a drug useful in the treatment of heart disease. (W-LRI)

First, usually he *thinks* he knows the structure of the new substance, but this must be verified or the correct structure found by careful and elaborate measurements. Second, assuming the structure is known, it becomes necessary, or at least highly desirable, to be sure that the compound is relatively pure. Many laboratories have had the disheartening experience of discovering highly interesting biologic activity in the first sample of a new compound only to find that later samples do not possess it. Presumably the activity was due to an undetected impurity that usually could not be discovered by further experimentation.

Even at this early stage, the synthetic chemist is given a great deal of help by another group—the development chemists. They prepare for him known organic compounds, not readily available commercially, that he wishes to use as intermediates in making new compounds. These compounds also undergo analytical and physical chemical study to establish identity and purity.

When new compounds are made, the next step is to test them in various biologic systems. It is desirable that the chemists and biologists collaborate in setting up the biologic screening program; this insures maximal understanding by both groups of the objectives and limitations of the overall research program. In a general way, the activities of the biology group can be classified into five areas. First, there is a set of procedures that are screens or primary evaluations. Usually an attempt is made to submit all new compounds to all available screens. But often manpower limitations prevent this, and selective screening must be done. As a rule, the first test made is the one requested by the chemist. It has been a common experience, however, to find that new compounds have entirely unpredicted activity—and sometimes this has led to the discovery of new types of drug.

The screens selected will vary widely between different research groups. First, they are designed to detect possible drugs in therapeutic areas that are of interest to company management. Second, the exact screen used reflects the best judgment of the biologists that it is predictive of clinical activity. This is not an easy judgment to make, because the animals used do not (except possibly in the case of some infectious diseases) have the clinical entities for which a therapeutic agent is sought. Third, the manpower available may, and usually does, limit the number of screens that can be set up.

If a compound is active in a screen, and is not obviously too toxic to study further, it is given a secondary evaluation. In it, the type of activity in the primary evaluation is studied in depth in order to find out whether it is real and of interesting magnitude. Many compounds found in a primary screen are not judged worthy of intensive study after this secondary evaluation. For example, a compound may lower the blood pressure of normal animals as determined in the primary screen. When, however, it is given daily to animals with experimental high blood pressure, it may very well have no useful effect at all.

If the compound is still interesting after this secondary evaluation, it is subjected to a broad pharmacologic (including, if indicated, microbiologic) and biochemical study. There are several objectives. An interesting analgesic, as an example, might not be useful if it also lowers blood pressure, or causes diarrhea, or makes the animal sleepy—or does any one of a number of things. If none of these undesirable effects is observed, biochemical studies are designed to find out how well the compound is absorbed, what happens to it in the body, and how it is excreted.

At some time during these activities, it is necessary to determine the degree of toxicity produced by the compound in different animal species. The types of study done will be described later in this chapter. Finally, a certain amount of what was described in Chapter 1 as basic research should be carried out by the biologists. This research is designed to obtain new biologic knowledge that will make it possible to devise new and meaningful biologic testing and evaluation procedures. This is one of the most essential and, unfortunately, often one of the most neglected activities of the biologists. It is an area from which it is tempting to "steal" manpower when the pressures generated by the desire to speed up the development of a potential new drug become great.

The biologic effort involves a number of specialists. The microbiology group always includes bacteriologists, and often virologists, mycologists (specialists in the study of fungi), and immunologists. The larger research groups may have parasitologists, interested in parasites such as intestinal protozoa, intestinal worms, and in diseases such as trichomonas vaginalis vaginitis, a common disorder of women.

Other scientists are physiologists (who study the various functions of the body), pharmacologists (who study the effect of drugs in the body), endocrinologists (who are specialists in the study of hormones), biochemists, toxicologists (who set up and carry out toxicity tests), and pathologists (who specialize in examining animals and tissues from them for evidences of tissue injury after toxicity testing). The large number of animals used, and the need to keep them reasonably healthy, makes it desirable to have one or more veterinarians on the staff.

The chemist, then, makes a new compound, establishes to his satisfaction that it has the proper structure and is reasonably pure, and submits it for biologic evaluation. Let us suppose that it has interesting activity in the primary screen, and that secondary evaluation suggests that it should be studied intensively. Now it becomes highly desirable to devise a careful plan involving several groups. If this is not done, the time required for development of the new agent (long enough under optimal conditions) probably will be lengthened considerably because procedures that could be carried out simultaneously will be done one after the other. This planning includes the following:

1. The pharmacologic (and microbiologic if indicated) and biochemical studies.

2. The toxicity testing required before study in man can be undertaken.

3. Work by the development chemists and chemical engineers, who must prepare sufficient quantities of the compound for the laboratory studies and for later clinical trials. Laboratory studies alone often require fifty pounds or more and the clinical studies may well require several hundred pounds, depending, of course, on the size of the clinical dose.

4. Studies by the pharmacists, who must later prepare dosage forms for use in the human studies and, if the trials are successful, for transfer to the production area. They are assisted by the pharmaceutical analytical group, who devise the assays required to show that the dosage forms contain the proper amount of compound and who assay these dosage forms at intervals to establish stability. Incidentally, stability studies usually are carried out with preparations that have been stored at several temperatures and at several ranges of relative humidity.

5. Plans for the writing of an informative brochure that will be supplied to clinical investigators if the agent is studied in humans.

6. The timing of the filing of necessary documents with the Food and Drug Administration prior to clinical testing.

7. The various phases of clinical testing.

8. The long-range toxicity program in animals.

9. Assembling all information into a New Drug Application to be submitted to the Food and Drug Administration when it is believed that enough work has been done to show that the drug is sufficiently safe and efficacious to justify marketing.

The toxicologists begin their studies by determining the LD_{50} (lethal dose fifty: the dose required to kill 50 percent of the animals) in four species of animal. Usually mice, rats, and dogs are used; the fourth species varies: it may, for example, be hamsters, guinea pigs, rabbits, or (rarely) monkeys. This measures the intrinsic toxicity of the compound and indicates whether it has unusual toxicity in one species of animal as compared to others. The toxicity studies carried out prior to clinical testing usually are done in rats and dogs. Before protocols can be set up for these tests, range-finding experiments must be done. That is, the toxicologist must attempt to find out how much drug can be given for a period of some days without killing the animal. Frequently, also, he will give large doses in the attempt to determine which organs may be damaged by an overdosage of the drug.

With this information, the toxicologist sets up his subacute (or preclinical) test protocols. Usually the compound is administered at three dosage levels to two groups of animals (rats and dogs). An attempt is made to adjust dosage so that the highest dose is toxic, and will give information of further value in predicting the effects produced if toxic doses should be given later to humans.

The period of administration of the agent will vary, depending on how it will be used in the clinic. If it is to be given to humans for a few days only (that is, if it is designed to be used in the treatment of an acute disorder), this period usually is one month. If a long period of treatment is anticipated, the usual period is three months. A typical "three-month" study actually requires a period of about six months to complete. The animals must be procured and conditioned prior to initiating the study, and numerous blood studies, urinalyses, and physical examinations are done. At the end of the period—and usually in the middle of it—blood and chemical tests are repeated. After the period of administration is over and the studies mentioned are completed, the animals are sacrificed and examined by the pathologist. Samples of many tissues are obtained and processed, after which they are studied microscopically by the pathologist.

If the initial clinical trials are promising, and it is a good bet that the compound will become a marketed drug, chronic (long-range) toxicity studies must be set up. The timing usually is such that at least three or more months of drug administration have been concluded before wide-scale administration to humans is undertaken. For some potential drugs (although admittedly procedures are changing), periods of administration of six months for dogs and one year for rats are used. If the drug is one that will be given to patients constantly for long periods of time, the usual periods are one year in dogs and eighteen months to two years in rats. As in the subacute studies, usually three levels of dosage are used, and careful studies of blood cells, blood chemistry, urinalysis, body weight, and physical examination and observation are carried out. Blood studies and urinalysis are done at three-month intervals for a year, and at six-month intervals thereafter. Again, careful pathologic studies are done and an "eighteen month" chronic study actually may require as long as two years, and even more if something goes wrong during the long period of experimentation.

These tests are expensive. It costs about $8 per month per

rat and $110 per month per dog to carry them out. The compound cannot be given to women of child-bearing age until other toxicity tests are completed. These tests, which require from six to eight months to complete, are designed to detect toxicity during gestation and lactation, to detect teratogenicity (tendency to produce physical abnormalities in the newborn), and adverse effects on conception. Two species of animal are used in carrying out the teratogenic tests. One of these ordinarily is the New Zealand white rabbit, one of the few animals useful in detecting the teratogenic potentiality of thalidomide, the compound that caused malformations in thousands of infants at the beginning of this decade. Either the rat or the mouse commonly is used for the other tests.

The total cost of a complete set of toxicity studies, assuming the eighteen-month study in rats and the one-year study in dogs, is approximately $150,000, assuming that no part of the experiments needs to be repeated and that no additional tests are required. In actual practice, the cost probably averages $250,000.

During the period of initial and subacute toxicity testing, the development chemists and the pharmacists have been busy. The development chemists must prepare the large quantities of compound required for the clinical trial—or at least enough to allow an adequate assessment of its probable clinical utility. If the drug is to be marketed, this group will work out a tentative method of production that will be sent on to the chemical production plant. The pharmacists must furnish the dosage forms needed in the clinic. Frequently the first clinical experiments are conducted with capsules of the powdered drug, but commonly other dosage forms, such as tablets, liquids, or ampules for injection will be requested. All of these must be checked analytically for both accuracy of dosage and for stability. In most cases, samples of the dosage forms are given to

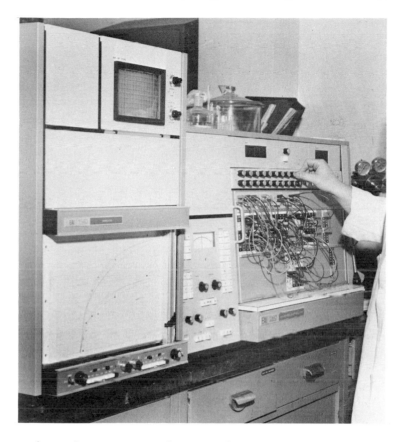

An analog computer. After certain chemical properties of a potential new drug have been determined in the laboratory, the computer can be used to predict how the new substance will behave in animals and in humans. (W-LRI)

animals to make sure that nothing toxic has become incorporated during their preparation.

When the preclinical toxicity studies have been completed,

everything known about the new agent—its chemistry, biology, toxicology, pharmacy, and research manufacturing and control procedures—is assembled and incorporated into a document known as a "Notice of Claimed Investigational Exemption for a New Drug"; the short term generally used in the industry is "IND," the letters derived from the words *Investigational New Drug*. This document also includes the qualifications of the key people who carried out the research and of the persons who decided it is reasonably safe to conduct clinical investigations. In addition, it must contain an outline of the plans for the clinical investigations, including the names and qualifications of the investigators who will conduct the studies. The completed IND is sent to the FDA (Food and Drug Administration). Legally it is possible to begin clinical investigations at this point, and sometimes this is done. Since, however, the FDA can stop an investigation if it does not believe the IND contains enough information to justify clinical studies, in many cases an informal discussion with the appropriate members of the FDA staff is held before the investigation begins.

The IND assumes that the clinical studies will be conducted in three phases. Phase 1 is a period of human pharmacology, in which investigations designed to indicate toxicity, dosage, absorption, excretion, and fate in the body are carried out. The subjects used may be healthy volunteers, although this is not a requirement. Phase 2 refers to limited trial of the new agent in patients who have the disorder that the drug is designed to treat, which will indicate its possible clinical utility. Phase 3 refers to a large-scale clinical trial in patients with the specific disease for which the new drug is indicated. In reality, these three phases merge and overlap, but in practice this presents no real difficulty.

Research groups in pharmaceutical companies usually do not have patients available to their clinical investigational staff, although a few groups have established arrangements in hospitals that make this possible to a limited extent. The actual investigations, then, are carried out by competent medical scientists throughout the United States, and for that matter, in other countries as well. The pharmaceutical clinical scientist works with the pharmaceutical statisticians in setting up a total meaningful study and with the individual investigators in devising suitable protocols. He sends out the clinical supplies and maintains close contact with each investigator as the studies proceed. He keeps the investigators informed of interesting findings or evidence of toxicity observed by others. Finally, he correlates (with the aid of the statisticians) the results of all of the investigations and, together with his superiors, evaluates the results. In a favorable situation the judgment will be that the drug is sufficiently safe and efficacious to justify marketing.

Before marketing, however, the FDA must agree that the data obtained do indeed justify it. A document known as a New Drug Application (NDA) is prepared and sent on. This contains full reports of both laboratory and clinical investigations. The laboratory data section of this document is more complete than that of the IND (including supplementary information, both from the laboratory and from the clinic, periodically sent to the FDA during the clinical studies) because pharmacologic, toxicologic, and biochemical investigations will have continued even after clinical trial has been initiated. Chemical and pharmaceutical data are included, as well as a description of the proposed manufacturing facilities, manufacturing procedures, and control procedures. The labeling is furnished, including the package insert and any descriptive brochures that will be used when the drug is marketed. Of course, complete clinical records accompany the NDA: the names of the investigators, detailed information regarding each patient subject studied, and adequate summaries and conclusions regarding the results obtained are included in the document.

The law provides that the FDA will reply within six months after receipt of an NDA, to indicate either approval or disapproval. In actual practice, this period often is extended by mutual agreement so that differences of opinion between the pharmaceutical group and the FDA can be ironed out. Often this requires additional work, usually in the clinic, but sometimes in other areas. For example, there may be a disagreement about the adequacy of a control procedure or the wording of the label or package insert. My own guess is that the time required for an NDA to be approved at the present time varies from about one year to about four years, with an average of two years. Recently the FDA has acknowledged that the "usual" period required is eighteen months, but the agency is optimistic that this period can be shortened in the near future.

If the new drug is an antibiotic, the NDA form is not used; instead, Antibiotic Forms 5 and 6 are sent. These forms include essentially the same information required for an NDA, but also (Form 5) request certification by the FDA of the new antibiotic. This means that the appropriate FDA laboratory will assay the antibiotic to determine that it has the required potency and safety, and that it meets certain other standards of quality. Even after the drug is on the market, each manufactured batch must be so certified, and Antibiotic Form 7 is used to request certification of each batch of a marketed antibiotic. Form 6 contains a complete description of the manufacturing and control procedures that will be used for the marketed drug.

It will be instructive for us to construct a time table. It will be assumed that the compound chosen has already been studied sufficiently to justify its development. Moreover, only the time-limiting procedures will be included—other necessary studies, it is assumed, can be proceeding simultaneously. Of course, these times will vary somewhat for each compound, but the figures given are typical. The schedule is conservative in the sense that it assumes everything proceeds smoothly, as, in actual practice, it seldom does. In other words, the actual time required for a given drug might be longer, sometimes much longer.

	Months
1. Time from submission by the chemist to completion of the screening test	3
2. First phase of secondary evaluation	6
3. First toxicity tests	3
4. Subacute toxicity	6
5. IND prepared and filed	3
6. Clinical studies, phase 1	9
7. Clinical studies, phase 2	12
8. Clinical studies, phase 3	21
9. Preparing and filing NDA	3
10. Approval of NDA by the FDA	24
Total time	*90 months* (*or* 7½ *years*)

CHAPTER *3*

Some Vignettes of Synthetic Drugs

Serendipitous or deliberate? A medical-student researcher
and many helpful drugs. Phenothiazine. Chlorpromazine
and the tranquilizers

It is fashionable to say that many of our most useful drugs
have been found by *serendipity*, the "faculty for making desirable discoveries by accident." I cannot quite go along here,
for the simple reason that the alert scientists in the pharmaceutical industry *are always looking* for new drugs, even if
they lurk in unexpected places. One particular type of chemical structure may yield several very different drugs, often
unexpectedly, it is true. But no unexpected new drug is
found unless someone, either in the laboratory or in the clinic,
observes the unusual biologic behavior that leads eventually to
the creation of a new therapeutic agent. When a chemist
makes a brand new type of chemical compound, there is no
way for him or for the biologist to know what type of biologic
activity, if any, it will possess. If indeed it is found to have a
useful type of activity, this might be cited as an example of
"finding what you are not looking for." This is not serendipity,
however, because it involves a purposeful search, not a blind,
lucky stumbling onto the usefulness of the new compound.

It is true enough that some of our best drugs have resulted
from the observation that they had unexpected biologic or
clinical activity. In other words, the activity actually observed
was not the activity hoped for when the new substance was
created. In other cases, of course, drugs have possessed the
activity hoped for at the moment of chemical creation. These
vignettes may illustrate these points.

42

When Paul Ehrlich was a medical student in Germany in the 1880s, he was intrigued by the phenomenon of vital staining. When certain dyes were injected into animals and their tissues later examined microscopically, subcellular structures in some cells were found to be stained, but not the whole cell. If, he reasoned, a dye could be found that would stain microorganisms but not animal tissues, and if this dye were toxic to the microorganisms, it might prove to be chemotherapeutic. In collaboration with the Japanese scientist, K. Shiga, he was successful in finding that trypan red, a complex dye, was active against trypanosomes in the animal body. This is the organism that causes a type of sleeping sickness in the tropics, especially in Africa. At one time, trypan red was used with some success in the treatment of trypanosomiasis. In 1910, working with another Japanese scientist, Dr. Hata, Ehrlich discovered arsphenamine (Compound 606, Salvarsan) and, later, the more useful neoarsphenamine. These yellow compounds were used for many years in the standard treatment of syphilis.

Some years later, two German chemists, Fritz Mietzsch and Joseph Klarer, intrigued by the earlier work of Ehrlich, prepared a number of dyes that were screened against pathogenic bacteria *in vitro* (literally "in glass"; i.e., not in the animal). Active compounds were found, but they did not prove effective in animals infected with disease-producing bacteria. They were working in the laboratories of I. G. Farbenindustrie in Wuppertal-Elberfield. Dr. Gerhard Domagk, a member of the faculty at the University of Münster, was a consultant. In 1929, the Company built a new research institute for pathologic anatomy and bacteriology, and Dr. Domagk became its head with the title, Director of the Institute of Experimental Pathology. He and the two chemists decided to discard *in vitro* testing in favor of *in vivo* ("within the living body") testing of all compounds against streptococcal infections in mice. The first active dye was found in 1931; it contained a chemical group known as a sulfonamide group. Soon after, in 1932, Domagk found that a dye (sulfamidochrysoidine hydrochloride), later known by the trademark, Prontosil Rubrum, protected both mice and rabbits against infections caused by hemolytic streptococci and staphylococci. The new agent had almost no activity *in vitro*. A German patent was applied for by Mietzsch and Klarer on December 24, 1932, and Domagk did not publish the results of his experiments until February 15, 1935, after the issuance of the German patent on January 2, 1935.

Domagk was not at all certain that this compound would be active in man. However, when his own daughter contracted a severe streptococcal infection, in desperation he gave her the drug, and she recovered completely. This episode was not mentioned in Domagk's first paper. Domagk was awarded the Nobel prize in 1939, but he was prevented from accepting it then because of the political situation in Germany. He received the coveted diploma and gold medal at a ceremony held finally in 1947.

A group of scientists working at the Pasteur Institute in Paris played a hunch that Prontosil Rubrum "came apart" in the animal, yielding, as one product, sulfanilamide. This chemical, although made in 1908 by the German scientist, P. Gelmo, had not been studied as a potential drug. Late in 1935, the husband and wife team, Trefouel and Trefouel, working with Mitti and Bovet, reported that sulfanilamide was as active as Prontosil Rubrum, and the modern era of chemotherapy began. Since 1935, more than twenty sulfa drugs have been marketed in this country. Some are most useful for acute systematic infections; others for activity in the gastrointestinal tract, activity in the urinary tract, for prophylaxis against attacks of rheumatic fever, for meningitis, and for even topical use in the eye. The original discovery has led to the development of a variety of agents useful in combating infection.

In 1940, T. Mann and D. Keilin reported in England that sulfanilamide was a powerful inhibitor of the enzyme carbonic anhydrase *in vitro*. Other scientists found that this inhibition occurred also in the animal body. On theoretical grounds, it was postulated that such a compound should increase the excretion of sodium salts from the body by way of the urine, which in turn should cause an increase in the volume of water excreted, since the sodium salts, of course, were dissolved in body water. These physiologic effects should be useful in treating a number of clinical syndromes in which there was a retention of sodium and water in the body. Among these were high blood pressure, cirrhosis (hardening) of the liver, and various kidney and heart diseases. Because sulfanilamide was found to have some activity in increasing the excretion of sodium in man, though not enough to make it a useful agent, the search for a useful compound began.

In 1953, the compound Diamox (the proprietary name used by Lederle Laboratories for the compound acetazolamide, which contained the sulfonamide group in its molecule) was marketed. It was useful medically, but since it was a powerful inhibitor of carbonic anhydrase everywhere in the body, including the red blood cells, it had side effects that made it ineffective after use for a few days. It was necessary, then, to space its use—that is, to use it for a few days, discontinue it for a few days, use it again, and so on. Meanwhile, a group of scientists at Sharp & Dohme (later Merck Sharp & Dohme) had been studying the problem. Instead of using the inhibition of carbonic anhydrase as an assay procedure, they measured the effect of experimental compounds on the kidney function of trained dogs. The first compound that seemed truly potent and relatively nontoxic in their tests was a great disappointment; it was not absorbed when it was given by mouth to humans. However, later the substance known as Diuril (Merck Sharp & Dohme's proprietary name for chlorothiazide) was discovered. It was a sulfonamide derivative, but interestingly enough it was only a weak inhibitor of carbonic anhydrase. Perhaps this explains why it did not possess some of the undesirable side effects of Diamox.

Diuril was marketed in 1958, and proved extremely useful in medicine. It caused a loss of sodium and water in many cases in which their abnormal storage in the body was a problem, and in addition, it soon became evident that it was useful in the therapy of high blood pressure, especially when it was given in conjunction with other agents for this purpose. About ten active drugs chemically related to Diuril now are on the market.

The scientists who discovered and developed Diuril had

Prominent members of the MS&D Laboratories, which discovered and developed Diuril—Drs. John Baer, Karl Beyer, Frederick Novello, and James Sprague. (MS&D)

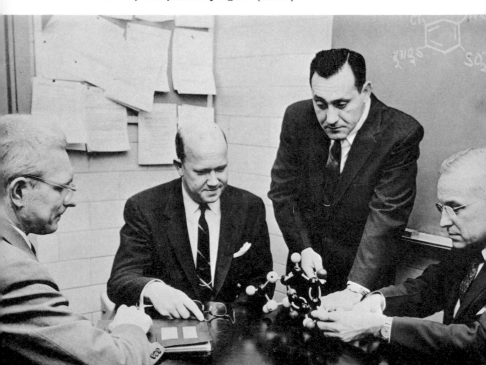

predicted that it would be useful in hypertension. It was known that the blood pressures of patients with hypertension could be lowered by giving them diets that were low in sodium, and it seemed reasonable to suppose that a drug that would cause a loss of sodium from the body would yield the same result. In spite of this plausible explanation, scientists in the Schering Laboratories tested various compounds related chemically to Diuril, but devoid of sodium-excreting properties. One of the compounds they studied, diazoxide, lowered blood pressure in animals and in patients with hypertension. It caused a *decreased* excretion of sodium in the humans, and in the first studies this unwanted effect was overcome by giving a compound, trichlormethiazide, that, like Diuril, caused an increased excretion of sodium. It soon became evident that this combination of agents caused an unexpected rise in blood sugar, resulting in symptoms similar to those of patients with diabetic coma. Further investigation showed that the diazoxide alone also caused a rise in blood sugar, presumably as a result of suppression of insulin production.

There is a clinical syndrome known as hypoglycemia,* in

* It was this illness that Esau was victim of, according to Robert B. Greenblatt, MD, a great endocrinologist, and which gave him so great a body need that he "sold" his birthright to Jacob for a "mess of pottage."

> And Jacob sod [boiled] pottage: and Esau came from the field, and he was faint:
> And Esau said to Jacob, Feed me, I pray thee, with that same red pottage; for I am faint: . . .
> And Jacob said, Sell me this day thy birthright.
> And Esau said, Behold, I am at the point to die: and what profit shall this birthright do to me?
> . . . and he sold his birthright unto Jacob.
> Genesis 25:29-33

Today, Esau might have recovered his well-being by taking a drug containing diazoxide—and held onto his valuable birthright.
From R. B. Greenblatt: *Search the Scriptures* MODERN MEDICINE AND BIBLICAL PERSONAGES (Philadelphia, Lippincott, 1968, Chapter 11, pp. 67ff.)

which the blood sugar is abnormally low. It has many causes, for example: overdosage of insulin, tumors of the pancreas, mushroom poisoning, sensitivity to leucine, an amino acid present in proteins, endocrine (hormonal) diseases, liver disease, and so on. Some of these conditions are acute, but others are chronic and crippling. The limited clinical studies carried out with diazoxide have shown the drug effective in lowering the blood sugar in all of these conditions. However, the compound produces side effects that probably will prevent its development as a therapeutic agent. The most obvious is a marked increase in the appearance and growth of body hair, not so evident in adult males but obvious in females and in children. The excess hair disappears several weeks after administration of the drug is stopped. Other troublesome side effects are retention of body water, vomiting, abdominal pain, loss of appetite, and rapid beating of the heart.

The importance of diazoxide is that it may lead to another compound that will be useful in the treatment of hypoglycemia. Although hypoglycemia is not widespread, a drug of this sort would be extremely important, in some cases life-saving, for patients with the chronic type. Patients with chronic hypertension sometimes have a hypertensive crisis—a life-threatening condition characterized by a marked increase in diastolic pressure—the lowest blood pressure during a heart beat. Usually this results from some stress situation, such as an infection or an emotional upset. An intravenous injection of diazoxide usually rapidly reduces the diastolic pressure for three to six hours. During this time the doctor can institute measures designed to prevent the return of the diastolic pressure to a dangerous level. Probably the drug will be marketed for this limited medical indication. If so, it can be classed with the drugs discussed in Chapter 11 as a "drug without profit."

Even before the discovery that sulfanilamide was a chemotherapeutic agent, Argentine scientists (C. L. Ruiz, L. L. Silva, and L. Libenson) had reported that several sulfonamide compounds caused a lowering of blood sugar. In 1942, M. Janbon, J. Chaptal, A. Vedel, and J. Schaap, working at the University of Montpellier in France, reported that patients undergoing experimental treatment for typhoid fever with the sulfonamide, isopropylthiodiazole, exhibited hypoglycemia (lowered blood sugar). During the period 1942-1946, A. Loubatieres, another scientist at the University of Montpellier, studied this phenomenon. He suggested that this type of compound, if sufficiently potent and nontoxic, might be useful in the treatment of patients with diabetes mellitus. He also furnished evidence that the mechanism of action was to speed the release of insulin from the pancreas.

German industrial scientists took up the study, and in 1956 Gustav Ehrhart, a chemist working in the laboratories of Farbwerke Hoechst, in Frankfurt, announced the synthesis of the compound now known as tolbutamide, marketed in this country in 1957 by Upjohn under their proprietary name, Orinase. The drug is especially useful in the treatment of mild diabetes in the older age group, which patient seems to have insulin in his pancreas but for some reason does not utilize it or secrete it normally. In types of diabetes in which the pancreas does not manufacture enough insulin (for example, in many cases of diabetes in children), it is not effective. In addition to Orinase, three other related drugs are on the United States market—chlorpropamide (Diabinese, Pfizer), acetohexamide (Dymelor, Lilly), and tolazamide (Tolinase, Upjohn).

A sulfonamide derivative, also, is another useful drug that was developed by the Sharp & Dohme laboratories. In 1943, penicillin was scarce, and the objective of the project was to find a drug that would keep penicillin in the body for longer periods of time, thus reducing the necessary clinical dose. As the blood flows through the kidney, some of the substances in it diffuse through a filter termed the glomerular membrane and into small tubules. These small tubules unite to form larger ones and eventually become the ureter, the tube that transports urine from the kidney to the urinary bladder. As the filtrate (material that has passed through the glomerular membrane) passes down the microscopically small tubule, some of the filtered substances diffuse through its walls and back into the blood. In some cases, however, the cells that line the tubules actually extract compounds from the blood and secrete them into the inside (lumen) of the tubules. Penicillin is such a substance; about one fifth of it is lost from the blood by glomerular filtration, and the other four fifths by tubular secretion.

The Sharp & Dohme scientists reasoned that it might be possible to find a compound that, like penicillin, was eliminated from the blood mainly by tubular secretion. Perhaps the tubular "pump" (mechanism) could be "filled up" by the substance so that it had no capacity left to secrete the penicillin. A compound used in studying kidney function, para-aminohippuric acid, was known to be secreted by tubular secretion, and was used in testing the hypothesis. It worked. It was not a practical drug, however, because it was necessary to give a patient about sixty grams (two ounces) daily by vein in order to prevent the tubular loss of penicillin.

The chemists at Sharp & Dohme had discovered several useful sulfa drugs and it was natural for them to seek the wanted drug in this area of chemistry. The first compound they found that was thought worthy of testing in humans was a sulfonamide derivative known as carinamide. It was active by mouth, but the dosage required was again excessive—about twenty grams (two thirds of an ounce) daily. Nevertheless, it was marketed for a time under the trademark, Staticin. Further work led to the discovery of another derivative, probenecid. This compound was combined with penicillin and the combination was marketed under the proprietary name, Remanden. By this time (approximately 1950), however, penicillin had become plentiful and cheap enough to make the combination product uneconomic, and it did not go far in the market place, although it is still listed in the Merck Sharp & Dohme catalogue.

One waste product secreted in the urine of humans is difficult to study in animals: uric acid, the end product of certain compounds found in every cell—the purines. Man, the higher apes, and the Dalmatian coachhound excrete this substance, and birds also, but most of the uric acid in the bird excreta comes from protein and only a small portion from purines. The way in which uric acid is excreted by the Dalmatian coachhound differs from the method of excretion in the human, and so this is not a useful animal to use in predicting the effect of a new drug on the elimination of uric acid by the human.

During the clinical testing of carinamide and, later, probenecid, it was found that these substances actually increased the elimination of uric acid in the urine, thus lowering the level of this substance in the blood. Now in the disease gout, at least at times, there is an increase in the level of uric acid in the blood, and this substance (or more properly its sodium salt) may precipitate as tiny crystals in the cartilage of joints. This is especially likely to happen in the big toe, but any joint may be involved. Involvement causes an extremely painful clinical episode. If such attacks continue to occur over a long period of time, gouty arthritis, characterized by permanent deposits of urate crystals (the resulting swollen areas are termed tophi) around joints, can result. Probenecid, marketed in 1951 under the trademark, Benemid, has proved useful in treating gout in much the same way that tolbutamide or insulin is useful in the treatment of diabetes mellitus. It must be taken every day, but usually it eliminates or reduces the number of acute attacks of gout, and under its administration over long periods of time the tophi of gouty arthritis frequently diminish in size or even disappear.

Thus the pioneering thoughts of a German medical student, long since dead, have resulted in a rich variety of potent and useful therapeutic agents.

ﻬﻪ ﺟﻪ

Phenothiazine was first synthesized by the German chemist, Bernthsen, in 1888. It became the parent substance from which various dyes were made. One of these was methylene blue, widely used as a stain in bacteriology. About 1935, it was used as an insecticide and as a vermifuge (agent to expel worms from the intestinal tract) in veterinary medicine, and it still is used for these purposes today. For a brief period it was thought useful in human medicine, both as a vermifuge and as a urinary antiseptic. In 1942 and 1943, a number of reports of toxicity appeared in the literature. The toxic effects—liver damage, destruction of red blood cells, rapid heart beat, abdominal cramps, blood in the urine—were serious and the use of the drug in human medicine was discontinued.

During the 1940s, the French firm, Rhone-Poulenc, made a number of derivatives of phenothiazine. The first of these to become a new drug, promethazine hydrochloride, was marketed in this country by Wyeth Laboratories in 1951 under their trademark, Phenergan. Phenergan was a potent, long-acting antihistamine, but it had other interesting activities as well. For one thing, it was a sedative and hence especially useful for nighttime administration to patients who had allergic conditions responsive to antihistamines. For another, it was an antinausea agent. In laboratory studies, and later in the clinic, it was found to enhance the sedative properties of barbiturates.

An interesting phenomenon, true not only of Phenergan but of other antihistamines as well, was the lack of observable sedative effect in animals. It seemed likely, however, that the potentiation of the sedative effects of barbiturates might be predictive of sedation in the clinic. Rhone-Poulenc decided to use this test in the search for other potential sedative compounds. Hexobarbital (then marketed under the proprietary name Evipal), a barbiturate that acted quickly and had a short duration of action, was chosen as the barbiturate. By 1951 the most active of all the compounds they tested, identified by their laboratory designation RP 4560, was chosen for more complete investigation. RP 4560 had a bewildering array of activities in the laboratory studies. It lowered body temperature, was a sedative, prevented vomiting induced by giving apomorphine, decreased the activity of the autonomic nervous system (the part of the nervous system that acts automatically without conscious control), and disrupted conditioned responses (automatic responses to a signal as a result of training). Moreover it potentiated the activities of sedatives, anesthetics, analgesics, and curare-like drugs (drugs that cause muscular paralysis).

The French anesthesiologist, H. Laborit, working in the Military Hospital in Paris, was interested in what he termed "artificial hibernation." In his first work, he lowered the body temperatures of patients who were to be subjected to anesthesia. Under these circumstances, the need for blood of the body tissues, especially the brain, was reduced, and the amount of anesthetic used could be decreased. Since RP 4560 potentiated the activity of anesthetics and lowered body temperature, he became interested in finding out whether the new compound might be useful in producing a "chemical hibernation" in his patients. Probably an experiment carried out in animals by an associate, A. Bérritte, increased this interest; Bérritte cooled rats to a point where they quickly died. When the experiment was repeated exactly, except that RP 4560 was given, the animals became unconscious but did not die, and recovered after normal body temperature was restored. Laborit believed his work indicated that the new agent indeed was useful as an adjunct to anesthetics. He devised a mixture of drugs, of which RP 4560 was one, that he called the "lytic cocktail." Rhone-Poulenc marketed the compound, now known as chlorpromazine hydrochloride, under their trademark, Largactil, for use in anesthesiology. Meanwhile, in 1952, the Frenchmen Pierre Deniker and Jean Delay had published a report indicating that chlorpromazine showed promise as a useful drug in psychiatry.

During 1950 and 1951, the American firm, Smith, Kline & French (SK&F) had exchanged some information about potential new products with Rhone-Poulenc. It was not until April of 1952, however, that the French offered the American firm an opportunity to study chlorpromazine. As it happened, SK&F scientists had been using the Evipal-potentiation test in the search for a nonbarbiturate sedative. They were studying a compound, SK&F 525-A, that seemed almost devoid of pharmacologic activity of its own, but that increased the effectiveness of Evipal and a variety of other drugs. Naturally they welcomed the opportunity to study the new compound.

SK&F's first studies convinced them that there was something unusual about the sedation produced by the drug, but this was only a clue that would have to be investigated in the clinic. Moreover, they had the problem of deciding which of its numerous activities might be of most interest to American clinicians (who were, by the way, not especially interested in the "lytic cocktail"). There was only one publication and some verbal reports about its potential usefulness in mental disease; most publications concerned its use in anesthesiology and surgery. SK&F decided to evaluate the drug clinically against nausea and vomiting, severe mental disturbances, milder emotional states, and itching. The first reports to come in made it obvious that chlorpromazine was far more effective against nausea than the older drugs.

Psychiatrists were hard to convince that any drug could do more than act as a sedative in psychotic diseases, and reports in this field came in rather slowly. Two preliminary reports did arrive in late 1953, and within the next six months studies were begun in several large mental hospitals. A Canadian study sponsored by Rhone-Poulenc was published in February; it helped stimulate interest in the new drug. By October of 1953, more than 800 cases were in SK&F's files, and it was obvious that Thorazine (the SK&F trademark for chlorpromazine hydrochloride) was useful in several clinical situations. At the same time, however, disturbing reports that toxic side effects occurred in some patients also became available. The first of these was jaundice, indicating a toxic effect on the liver. Other side effects included a parkinsonian-like syndrome (a disorder in which the patient has severe muscular incoordination), gastrointestinal ulceration, and sensitivity to light. This picture made it appear desirable to recommend the use of the drug only in seriously ill patients.

Thorazine was marketed in the United States for the treatment of nausea and vomiting and for psychiatric use in May of 1954, two years and 3,000 patients after Rhone-Poulenc first told SK&F about RP 4560. (Such speed would be impossible today!) Thus was born a new type of synthetic drug, the tranquilizer. Clinically, this new drug produced a powerful sedative effect without the clouding of consciousness that occurs when sedation is produced by drugs such as barbiturates. In the laboratory, animals sedated with chlorpromazine are aroused easily; if they are held back-down above a flat surface and dropped, they turn over and land on their feet. Moreover, many times the dose that produces complete lack of physical activity can be given without apparent toxicity. In the case of some barbiturates, administration of as little as four times the sedative dose will produce death.

Thorazine does not cure severe mental disease, such as schizophrenia, but the effects it produces on such patients is nothing less than spectacular. Patients who paced in rooms with no furniture to smash or toilets to stuff with rags or clothes, who tore at the plaster on the walls, glared and shouted at nothing real—became calm and manageable. Other patients who lived so deeply within their own private dream worlds that communication was impossible became accessible, so that psychiatric treatment could be carried out. Many patients became well enough adjusted to return to their homes, and in 1956, the first time in 175 years, the number of patients in United States mental hospitals decreased. In 1955, the population of mental hospitals in this country was 633,505; in 1965, it had declined to an estimated 550,720. Nor does this tell the whole story. The number of mental patients undergoing treatment in outpatient clinics *increased* from 181,034 in 1959 (figures for previous years are not available) to 441,000 in 1965. Many of these patients would have been added to the hospital population if the potent tranquilizers had not been discovered and made available to the medical profession. By the end of 1963, 34 synthetic tranquilizers of varying degrees of potency were being marketed in the United States, and the number continues to grow. Some of these are not potent enough to be useful in serious mental disease, but they are sufficiently potent and free of toxicity to be useful in the management of the psychoneurotic disorders that plague so many Americans.

Dr. Leo H. Sternbach, presently employed with Hoffmann-La Roche as Director of Medicinal Chemistry, received his master's degree in pharmacy in 1929 and the PhD degree in chemistry in 1931 from the University of Cracow, Poland. As a research assistant there, he became interested in a readily accessible, little explored group of compounds known by the tongue-twisting name, heptoxdiazines. This interest resulted in several papers that were published together with his professor, K. Dziewonski, in the *Journal of the Polish Academy of Sciences* in the years 1933-35. Dr. Sternbach came to this country in 1941 as a member of the Hoffmann-La Roche chemical research team, and in the search for new types of compounds that might have interesting biologic properties, had the opportunity to return to the studies he had abandoned when he left Poland. The investigations were resumed in the 1950s, and led to the unexpected finding that these compounds had a different structure from that formerly postulated. Further

Naturally vicious cynomolgus monkeys are hostile to man and dangerous to handle: here, a control monkey attacks the handler's glove. After 2.5 mg/kg Librium (chlordiazepoxide HCl), the monkey is docile but alert: his aggression has declined by 75% of control, his activity by only 27%. (H-LAR INC.)

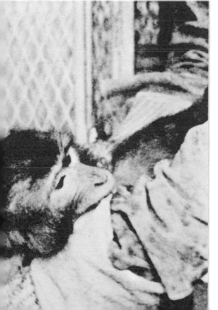
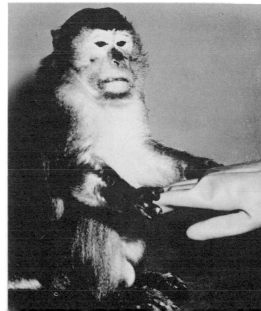

chemical transformations led ultimately in 1957 to the synthesis of the substance now known as Librium (Roche Laboratories' proprietary name for chlordiazepoxide hydrochloride). This type of chemical had never been tested in biologic systems, and it was impossible to anticipate what activity, if any, it might have. Nevertheless, Dr. Sternbach seems to have had that quality of insight so well developed in the best medicinal chemists. Playing a hunch, when he sent the new compound to the pharmacologists for testing he suggested that it might have activity in the central nervous system. Sure enough, it seemed to have tranquilizing activity similar to that of chlorpromazine, but without blocking the autonomic nervous system. When it was given to wild monkeys, they became, to all intents and purposes, tame animals, and could be handled with no difficulty. It had anticonvulsant properties resembling those of phenobarbital, but it was not a hypnotic (did not induce sleep).

The clinical staff at Roche made the new agent available to physicians for study after appropriate toxicity studies indicated that it was safe to do so. However, two other potential psychoneurotic compounds of more conventional chemical structure also were undergoing clinical study. The clinical investigators were urged to emphasize these two compounds at the expense of Librium, but things just did not work out that way. Without exception, they reported that Compounds A and B were of limited value, whereas Librium invariably produced impressive clinical results. Usually it is necessary for a pharmaceutical company to solicit the interest of clinical investigators in one of their new potential drugs. In this case, however, the medical grapevine was highly effective and Roche literally was flooded with requests from clinical investigators who wished to study Librium.

Studies also were carried out at the San Diego Zoo. Librium

was found to have a remarkable taming effect on a variety of wild animals—a Russian lynx, a Sumatra tiger, Australian dingos, marmosets, and other animals. Though tame, the treated animals were wide awake, playful, and cooperative. Roche made a movie at the Zoo that proved helpful in promoting the new drug when it was marketed.

Marketed in 1960, Librium has proved most useful in the management of patients with a variety of psychoneurotic (as opposed to psychotic) states. As a generality, it is useful whenever fear, anxiety, and tension are significant features of the disorder, and is especially valuable in the treatment of chronic alcoholism. Literally millions of patients have received Librium, and, from a commercial point of view, the drug has proved one of the most important ever marketed. Valium (Roche Laboratories' trademark for diazepam) is a second compound from Dr. Sternbach's series that has been marketed (in 1963) by Roche. Its clinical indications are very much the same as those for Librium, but, perhaps surprisingly, it too has become a popular drug.

The story of Librium underlines the value of making novel chemicals, even when no knowledge of their potential biologic activities exists.

CHAPTER 4

Drugs from Nature

The Vitamins. Aspirin. Salicin. Course of Development.
Vitamin B_{12} and APF. *Rauwolfia:*
reserpine. Antibiotics

U NTIL COMPARATIVELY RECENTLY, most useful drugs have been derived from natural sources. A few of them—for example, mercury, arsenic, and sulfur—were minerals. The most useful ones, however, were derived from plants, and familiar examples of such drugs, still used in therapy, are quinine, morphine, atropine, and digitalis. In the second quarter of this century, drugs of animal origin became important: the hormones and the enzymes. The vitamins were isolated from plant, animal, and microbial sources; and the antibiotics came from microorganisms.

For a while, it was hoped that the availability of the vitamins might make it possible to create potent antimicrobial drugs. The idea was to modify the vitamin chemically so that, although it still would attach itself to the sites in the bacteria that required it, it would not have activity. Since the site of attachment thus would be blocked, active vitamins could not reach it, and the bacteria would be injured or killed because of the resulting vitamin deficiency. This idea has not given us useful drugs, however, primarily because animals or humans receiving such compounds also react with signs suggesting severe acute vitamin deficiency. In other words, the antivitamins are too toxic to be useful, although a few of them have been used in the desperate attempt to treat cancer. With the hormones, chemical modification has been more successful, and most of the compounds having hormonal activity and that are used as drugs are derivatives of the hormones that exist in nature. Indeed, some of them bear little resemblance chemically to the hormone, although they possess the same qualitative activity.

ᥫᦲ ᦲᥫ

The most famous case in which a natural substance has been modified chemically to give a useful synthetic drug is that of aspirin. This drug probably is the most widely used, and the single most valuable, medicament in the world. In 1965, 29,089,000 pounds were produced in the United States. The bulk chemical had a monetary value of $14,380,000; and of course this figure is only a fraction of the money actually spent by the consumer for its various dosage forms at the retail level.

Thomas Sydenham,* a famous English physician of the seventeenth century, made it fashionable to search for remedies in the barks of trees. He was impressed by the medicinal properties of the bark of the cinchona tree, often called Peruvian or Jesuit's bark, which contained quinine. He found that the barks of the willow and the poplar yielded extracts that could reduce fever. Moreover, they had a bitter taste, which was regarded as an important property of potent drugs in those days.

The Reverend Edward Stone, in communications to the Royal Society in 1763, suggested the use of the willow tree to treat ague (fever and chills), though he did not mention Sydenham, and quite possibly did not know of his work. His account of his reason for using the willow bark is most inter-

---

* Philadelphians should know Thomas Sydenham, 1624-1689, for it has a Syndenham Street, with many charming homes on it. He practiced medicine in London, and his studies established him as a founder of modern clinical medicine and of epidemiology.

esting, although this method of finding new drugs is not in fashion today.

> As this tree delights in a moist or wet soil, where agues chiefly abound, the general maxim that many natural maladies carry cures along with them or that their remedies lie not far from their causes was so very apposite to this particular case that I could not help applying it; and that this might be the intention of Providence here, I must own, had some little weight with me.

In 1826, Brugnatelli and Fontana announced that the active principle of willow bark was a compound to be known as salicin, and Leroux isolated it in pure form in 1829. The Glasgow physician, MacLagan, began clinical work with salicin in 1874 and published his observations on its effectiveness in eight cases of rheumatic fever in 1876. He did not refer to the work of Stone, but then he was searching for a remedy for rheumatic disease rather than one to treat agues. His reasons for choosing a chemical derived from the bark of the willow were reminiscent of those given earlier by the Reverend Mr. Stone.

> It seemed to me that a remedy for that disease would most hopefully be looked for among those plants and trees whose favorite habitat presented conditions analogous to those under which the rheumatic miasma seemed most to prevail. A low-lying damp locality, with a cold rather than a warm climate, gives the conditions under which rheumatic fever is most readily produced. On reflection, it seemed to me that plants whose haunts best corresponded to such a description were those belonging to the natural order *Salicaceae*, the various forms of willow. Among the *Salicaceae*, therefore, I determined to search for a remedy for acute rheumatism. The bark of many species of willow contains a bitter principle called salicin. This principle was exactly what I wanted.

MacLagan first took a dose of the powder and, when it did not appear to be toxic, gave it to a patient. It gave relief to this first patient, seen on the fourth day of his second attack of rheumatic fever.

Some years earlier, the Swiss pharmacist Pagenstecher obtained the compound known as salicylaldehyde by distilling the flowers of the willow, *Spirea ulmaria*. He told the chemist Löwig about this, and in 1835 Löwig prepared salicylic acid from salicylaldehyde by means of a chemical process known as oxidation. Piria prepared salicylic acid from salicin in 1838, and in 1852, Gerland made salicylic acid by a completely synthetic process (not starting with a natural material). It was not until 1874, however, that a process suitable for commercial production was worked out by Kolbe and Lautemann. In 1877, a year after the publication of MacLagan's work with salicin, the German, Senator, suggested that salicylic acid in the form of its sodium salt might be active and less irritating; this proved true, and sodium salicylate became the drug of choice in the treatment of rheumatic disease.

Although sodium salicylate was less irritating than salicin, it caused gastric irritation in a number of patients and it had an unpleasant taste. In attempts to overcome these disadvantages, several other substances—among them salol, phenetsal, and salicylamide—were tried clinically, but none of them supplanted sodium salicylate. Then, late in the century, the story goes, the father of a chemist, F. Hoffmann, who worked in the chemical plant of Beyer, in Elberfeld, Germany (where Prontosil Rubrum was discovered later), asked his son to try to find a compound related to sodium salicylate that would not be as irritating as that drug. This man suffered from arthritis; and although sodium salicylate gave him relief, he was unable to tolerate it for long periods at a time. Back in 1853, von Gerhardt had prepared a derivative of salicylic acid known as acetylsalicylic acid. When this compound was tried in the clinic, it was found effective with minimal irritation; it was introduced to the medical profession in 1899 by Wohlgemut and by Dreser. Beyer marketed it under its trademark, Aspirin, a name suggested by the fact that the salicylic acid prepared from *Spirea nemaria* originally had been named acidum spiricum.

Aspirin was first widely used to supplant sodium salicylate, especially in the treatment of the rheumatic diseases. It was not long before its analgesic properties were recognized. Its greatest use then became that of the relief of pain, particularly muscular aching and headaches, although even today it is one of the drugs most useful in the management of the various forms of arthritis. In Germany and some other countries, Aspirin still is a valid trademark. In other countries, however—notably France, the British Commonwealth, and the United States—aspirin is a generic name and can be used by anyone.

>§ §≈

The course of development of a natural drug is similar to that outlined for a synthetic drug in Chapter 2. It might be argued that it would not be anticipated that substances such as vitamins and hormones, occurring normally in our bodies, would be toxic and that studies designed to show toxicity would be superfluous. Yet such studies were necessary during the development of the vitamins and the true natural hormones. Some of the vitamins, notably A, C, and D, have been given in dosages much larger than would be required for simple replacement of a lack in the diet, and this has necessitated special toxicity studies. For the hormones, two considerations are important reasons for searching for possible toxicity. First, most of the therapeutic agents in this field are not really hormones (since, by definition, a hormone is made in the body) but are substances having the biologic activities of the hormones. Second, some of them are used therapeutically in ways contrary to their normal physiologic use. For example, the famous contraceptive tablets are used in such a way that ovulation (expulsion of an egg from the ovary) is *prevented.* The natural hormones, having the same types of activities as the compounds present in the tablets, are secreted in a rhythmic fashion in the body so that normally ovulation *does* occur once each month. Patients with rheumatoid arthritis usually produce enough of the hormones of the adrenal cortex to supply physiologic needs. But if large doses (from a normal physiologic point of view) are given of these hormones, or of synthetic compounds having similar biologic properties, the symptoms of the arthritis often can be lessened. Here the compounds really are not being used as hormones but as synthetic therapeutic agents.

Dr. Thomas Addison, working at Guy's Hospital, London, identified and described the disease known as pernicious anemia in 1855, which disease is characterized by a deficiency in the number of circulating red blood cells. Those present are abnormally large. It is a slowly developing disease so far as the patient is concerned: usually he first notices a loss of weight; then weakness comes on; and, in 40 percent of the patients, signs of impairment of the spinal cord appear. These latter patients note tingling and numbness of the extremities; difficulty in walking, especially in the dark; and stiffness of the arms and legs. Patients who are not treated adequately die in two or three years after the appearance of the signs and symptoms of the disease. Laboratory studies during life indicate that these patients, in contrast to normal people, have no hydrochloric acid in their stomachs, and at autopsy, this finding is easily explained: the lining of the stomach is atrophied (wasted away) and thus incapable of producing its normal secretions.

Prior to 1926, about 6,000 Americans died of pernicious anemia each year. But in 1926, Minot and Murphy, working at Harvard University, found that adding one half to one pound of lightly cooked liver to the diet each day kept patients alive and in reasonably good health. In 1929, Castle, also at Harvard, found that the gastric content of normal people who were digesting meat also was effective. Further work made it evident that two substances were important: one was present in the diet, and termed the *extrinsic factor;* the other, which somehow facilitated the absorption of the extrinsic factor from the intestinal tract, was produced by the stomach, and was termed the *intrinsic factor.* The primary defect in pernicious anemia was a failure of the patient's stomach to produce sufficient intrinsic factor to permit absorption of the extrinsic factor in the food. Since liver was effective, evidently sufficient extrinsic factor was absorbed in spite of the deficiency of intrinsic factor if large enough amounts were given. In time, potent extracts of liver were developed that could be given by injection, thus obviating the need for intrinsic factor.

Although pernicious anemia was not a widespread disease, scientists at Merck decided to try to isolate the extrinsic factor, and began work on the problem in 1938. Dr. Karl Folkers, the chemist who headed the project, explained his interest in the problem in this way: "I had a hunch that if we ever identified a substance so fundamental to life as this compound was bound to be, it would prove to have more than enough completely unsuspected uses to justify all the patient persistence we would have to devote to finding it." At first, the going was slow and difficult. The disease could not be reproduced in animals, and preparations actually could be tested for activity only in patients with the disease who were not under treatment with liver extract. Only about one suitable patient could be located each month, even in populous New York City. And then came the break. Dr. Mary Shorb, a scientist working at the University of Maryland, had found a bacterium whose growth was promoted by liver extracts containing the extrinsic factor. It seemed probable, although not certain, that the factor responsible for this was in fact the extrinsic factor. Merck began to support her work, and it soon became evident from her tests that extracts useful in treating pernicious anemia were active, whereas clinically inactive extracts did not stimulate the growth of her bacterium. Merck scientists began to use the new rapid assay to detect activity in their liver fractions.

A search also was started for a source of extrinsic factor (as determined by the bacterial assay) that was cheaper and more abundant than liver. After many failures, it was found that one of the fermentation broths under study in the antibiotic laboratory was an excellent source. This broth resulted from the production of an antibiotic, grisein, discovered by Dr. Selman Waksman at Rutgers University. Then the next lucky break. The scientists who were carrying out the isolation studies observed the appearance of a pinkish color in extracts that had activity. As the extracts were concentrated, the depth of color seemed to parallel the increase in potency. The chemists now could proceed rapidly, simply by following the color of the fractions. On December 11, 1947, bright red crystals formed in a test tube containing a highly potent fraction of the factor. Nine days later, another member of the team produced identical red crystals from liver, and the story was almost complete. The final and clinching step was to test the red crystals in a patient with untreated pernicious anemia. Finding a proper patient required an exasperating two months of searching. At last, on February 21, 1948, an almost invisible amount of the red substance was injected into a suitable patient. Within five days, her body was making normal, new red blood cells at a rapid rate, and she became free of symptoms of the disease a few weeks later.

Since the new substance was required in trace amounts in the diet, it was by definition a vitamin. It was named vitamin B_{12}, and its official chemical name became cyanocobalamin. The red color apparently was caused by the fact that the metal, cobalt, was present in its molecule. Another clinically active form of the vitamin is known chemically as hydroxycobalamin; it is marketed by Merck under the trademark, alphaRedisol. Vitamin B_{12} is probably the most active of all known drugs. An amount as small as one microgram (about one thirty-millionth of an ounce) injected once monthly has been sufficient to maintain in a normal state some patients with pernicious anemia. Since the compound is harmless, and since patients vary in their requirement of it, the usual monthly maintenance dose is 100 micrograms. In animals, vitamin B_{12} is required for normal growth, and some physicians have used it in the treatment of growth failure in children. Some anemias other than true pernicious anemia respond to it; it has been used also as a supplement for animal feeds.

◄§ ۞►

The work done by Merck—in Rahway, New Jersey—was not the only search for the elusive red vitamin. In the research laboratories of Sharp & Dohme (S&D later merged with the Merck organization to form the present Merck Sharp & Dohme (MS&D) Research Laboratories), in Glenolden, Pennsylvania, an attempt was being made to isolate the factor, although at the beginning of the project it was not realized by either team that both were looking for the same substance. This story illustrates how a research project, even though it may be concluded successfully, can fail to lead to a product. The usual explanation is that a competitive organization won the race.

In 1942, S&D sent some pancreatic residue (left over from the production of insulin) to Dr. Abraham White, then a member of the Physiological Chemistry Department of Yale University. Dr. White was looking for a protein of good nutritional quality to use in making clinically useful digests of protein (protein hydrolysates) to be given intravenously to patients who needed protein, but who could not take it in adequate quantity by mouth. He reported that the pancreatic residue apparently contained a growth factor for rats, since they grew more rapidly when fed the pancreatic material than they did when the protein of the diet was furnished by soy bean protein or by casein (the principal protein of cow's milk). Since 1929 various investigators had noted that laboratory animals, especially rats and chicks, grew more rapidly when the protein of their diets was derived from animal sources rather than from plants. Sources as diverse as animal flesh, liver, fish meal, chicken droppings, cow dung, and fish solubles contained the factor, which became known as the animal protein factor, or APF. It was assumed both by Dr. White and by the scientists at S&D that the growth-stimulating factor in the pancreatic residue was APF.

The scientists at S&D repeated Dr. White's experiments, using, however, mice rather than rats as test animals. The first results were negative; the mice grew just as rapidly when fed casein as they did when fed the pancreatic residue. Examination of the diets used in the two laboratories soon explained this: the diet used at S&D contained a liver supplement, Dr. White's diet did not. When the liver supplement was omitted, the S&D mice grew faster on the pancreatic residue.

In 1946, S&D biochemists undertook the job of isolating the APF. At first, liver was used as a source of the new factor and the growth rate of mice served as a bioassay. The animal studies were too time-consuming to permit rapid progress, and the project was speeded up when a microbiologic assay was developed. Also, the liver was discarded in favor of the broth resulting from the growth of a soil bacterium that was being studied by the Antibiotics Department. As the isolation work proceeded, the pink color of active extracts made it seem likely that APF might be identical with the antipernicious anemia factor that the Merck scientists were purifying. Indeed, in late 1948, when crystalline APF was obtained at S&D, it proved identical with the vitamin B_{12} earlier isolated in Rahway. Thus, this very extensive effort did not lead to a product for S&D, but it did yield valuable scientific information that helped to solve the riddle of the animal protein factor. Merck and S&D later merged, and so vitamin B_{12} would have remained in the family regardless of which team won the race.

◄§ ◊►

For centuries, extracts prepared by immersing the roots of the snakeroot plant (*Rauwolfia serpentina*) in boiling water had been used in India as a "cure" for insanity. During the 1930s, some Indian physicians, trained in Western medicine, began reporting that the root of the plant was useful in treating high blood pressure. By the 1940s, Indian physicians had treated thousands of patients with both high blood pressure and mental disease with *Rauwolfia*. One of these was Dr. Rustom Jal Vakil, of Bombay. He published an account in English of his experiences with the drug in the treatment of patients with high blood pressure. As a result of reading this paper, Dr. Robert Wilkens of Boston University became interested in the drug. In 1952, Dr. Wilkens and his associates published a paper in which they concluded that snakeroot was indeed a useful drug in the treatment of hypertension (high blood pressure). In 1953, Squibb marketed tablets of the whole root of *Rauwolfia serpentina* (trademarked Raudixin) and Riker marketed a mixture of the alkaloids (complex nitrogen-containing compounds) extracted from the root. The Riker trademark was Rauwiloid.

During World War II, Dr. Emil Schlittler, a chemist employed by the CIBA Corporation of Basle, Switzerland, became interested in the Indian snakeroot; an authority on plant alkaloids, he had a special interest in colored alkaloids, and one of the alkaloids reported to be in snakeroot was serpentine, which was yellow. However, supplies of the plant could not be obtained at that time, and it was several years later before Dr. Schlittler and his group could work with *Rauwolfia*. When supplies did become available, Dr Schlittler, now also an Assistant Professor of Chemistry at the University of Basle, asked one of his graduate students to isolate serpentine. This was done, and a chemical explanation for the yellow color was worked out. Another compound, cryptolepine, of a deep purple color was purified and its structure determined. The next alkaloid isolated by the group was ajmaline, which produced a deep red color with nitric acid. Sir Robert Robinson, the famous English chemist who had been Dr. Schlittler's teacher, was interested in studying the structure of this substance, and large quantities of it were isolated and sent to him.

At this point, almost as an afterthought, Dr. Schlittler remembered the old reports he had seen on the sedative action of *Rauwolfia* extracts. Extracts prepared in his laboratory gave equivocal results when they were tested in animals, but fortunately, large quantities of mother liquors left from the isolation of serpentine, cryptolepine, and especially ajmaline had been saved, and when samples of these materials were injected into small animals, definite sedative effects were produced. The active alkaloid present in them was isolated and its structure was determined. It was named reserpine, and was marketed in this country by CIBA in 1953 under its trademark, Serpasil.

Dr. Schlittler and his wife were two of the first humans to take the new drug. When they swallowed the reserpine together at bedtime, he assured her they should have an excellent night's sleep. They stayed awake most of the night, waiting vainly for the expected hypnotic effect. Later experience in the clinic indicated that the effect expected by Dr. Schlittler did not occur until the patients had been receiving the drug orally for several days: immediate effects could be produced, but only if the drug were injected.

Clinical studies indicated that reserpine was useful in the treatment of hypertension, especially when it was given in combination with other antihypertensive drugs. It gave favorable effects also in some patients with such mental diseases as schizophrenia, paranoid and manic states, tertiary syphilis with psychosis, alcoholism, and even some depressions. Like Thorazine, reserpine had serious side effects in some patients. Usually therapy is stopped some time before surgery, because the combination of anesthesia and reserpine may result in a serious drop in blood pressure and in a slowing of the heart beat. It causes an increased secretion of acid in the stomach, an effect that is undesirable in persons with peptic ulcer. In rare cases, patients with psychiatric disorders develop a so-called parkinsonian syndrome with tremors, excessive secretion of saliva, muscular incoordination, and mental confusion; lethargy, nasal stuffiness, and difficulty in breathing may occur.

Several chemical derivatives of reserpine have been synthesized and marketed as drugs in this country. Their clinical properties are similar to those of reserpine.

∾§ §∾

The first antibiotic to be marketed in the United States was tyrothricin. It had been discovered by Dr. René J. Dubos, a member of the Rockefeller Institute, now Rockefeller University. Actually, as first marketed, it was a mixture of several substances, the most important of which were gramicidin and tyrocidine, and it was first introduced into veterinary medicine as an agent to treat mastitis (inflammation of the mammary glands) of cattle. When the agent was injected into the body, it caused hemolysis (disintegration of red blood cells), and so its use was limited to topical application. It was introduced into human medicine by S&D in 1942, and used in topical preparations—such as lozenges, nose drops, ointments, and solutions used to irrigate wounds and for instillation into the urinary bladder. It is used only rarely today. Like the penicillin marketed later, it was useful in treating infections caused by bacteria that are stained a deep violet (gram positive bacteria) by a method of staining developed by Gram. (Gram-negative bacteria develop a pink or red color when stained by this procedure.)

∾§ §∾

One day in 1928, a Scottish microbiologist named Alexander Fleming opened a culture plate (a small glass dish containing solidified agar and materials required as food by bacteria) on which staphylococci were growing. It had been left exposed to the air for a time, and when observed later, it was evident that a

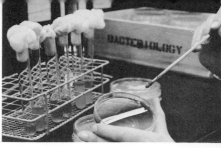

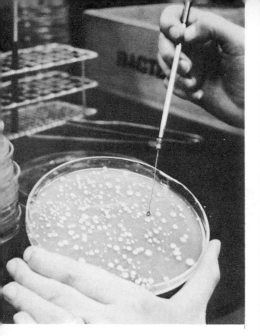

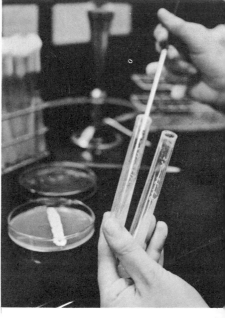

First steps in searching for a useful antibiotic. Promising mold cultures on soil plate are separated for study and testing. Six common disease microorganisms are smeared on streak plate to test effectiveness of the culture. Cultures that pass the streak test are transferred to agar-filled test tubes ("slants") for further study. (BL)

green mold had drifted into the room through an open window, settled on the surface of the plate, and grown into a readily observable green colony. The observation that excited Dr. Fleming was that the staphylococci in its vicinity were showing signs of dissolution.

Some of the mold spores were transferred to sterile agar plates and allowed to grow at room temperature for four or five days. Then different pathogenic bacteria were streaked onto the same plate. Some of them (the gram-negative ones) grew up to the mold colony, but the growth of others (the gram-positive bacteria) was inhibited for a considerable distance from the mold. Thus it seemed that the mold was manufacturing a substance that could diffuse through the agar and inhibit the growth of gram-positive bacteria. Dr. Fleming inoculated the mold into liquid growth media and found that it grew on the surface; under these circumstances it had an intense yellow color. When culture media containing the mold were injected into small animals, they were not more toxic than sterile media.

Then followed a frustrating twelve years, during which time the sulfa drugs were introduced into medicine. Dr. Fleming simply could not find a chemist who could, or would, purify the material and prepare enough of it so that it could be tried in human patients. Finally, on August 24, 1940, Florey and Chain, the Oxford chemists, together with a young assistant named Heatley, announced that they had prepared enough concentrated material to treat twenty five mice that had been given lethal doses of streptococci. Twenty four of the mice survived. During this same year, they tried to use the limited material they had to treat a patient suffering from septicemia but there was not enough drug and the patient died. In 1942, Fleming treated a middle-aged man suffering from streptococcal meningitis. He seemed to be dying in spite of treatment with sulfa drugs. After a few days of treatment with injections of the new agent, the patient made an uneventful recovery.

It was obvious that development of penicillin on a massive scale was needed if it was to become available as a therapeutic agent. Two of the British scientists came to the United States and presented their story to the government's wartime science agency as well as to a number of pharmaceutical companies; as a result of their efforts, a cooperative developmental program was undertaken. It involved laboratories in the Department of Agriculture and several American firms, notably Merck,

Pfizer, and Squibb. The truly massive effort included research, development, clinical testing, and a study of suitable production procedures. As a result, penicillin became available in limited amounts for the armed forces of the Allied Nations in 1943. During the last few months of 1943 and 1944, extremely small amounts of penicillin were allocated to United States citizens in accordance with decisions of an advisory committee under Dr. Chester Keefer. Later on, in 1945, there was general distribution of penicillin on an allocation basis for civilians within the United States. It is fair to state that the emergence of penicillin—discovered in Great Britain, developed by the United States government and pharmaceutical industry—was of more importance than any battle fought in World War II.

The story of penicillin illustrates the importance of chance observations in the laboratory that can lead to the discovery of therapeutic agents. Obviously these chance observations become important only if those scientists who make them have the wisdom to pursue the leads thus opened. Beyond a doubt, many scientists before Fleming had observed contamination of their bacterial plates by molds that produced clear zones around them. Probably they regarded this as a nuisance, perhaps a ruined experiment, rather than as an exciting discovery. As a matter of fact, the phenomenon of antibiosis—the inhibition of growth of one microorganism by another—had been observed in 1878 by the great French scientist, Louis Pasteur, who found that certain bacteria antagonized the growth of the anthrax organism.

⊰ ⊱

The word "antibiotic" was coined by Dr. Selman A. Waksman in 1941 and defined as "a chemical substance produced by microorganisms, which has the capacity to inhibit the growth and even to destroy bacteria and other microorganisms in dilute solution." Dr. Waksman discovered streptomycin, an antibiotic that was marketed in 1945, which had activity against gram-negative bacteria and proved to be especially useful in the treatment of tuberculosis. As subsequent events proved, the time was ripe for the discovery of a single antibiotic that would have activity against both gram-positive and gram-negative bacteria—in other words, a "wide spectrum" antibiotic.

In 1943 Dr. Benjamin M. Duggar, professor of botany at the University of Wisconsin, retired at age 72—not because he wanted to, but because a state law required retirement after age 71. Some of Professor Duggar's former students were working in the research laboratories at Lederle Laboratories. Lederle evidently believed that his experience with molds would be invaluable in their antibiotic research program. He happily accepted a position as a consultant in the research division. When he arrived, however, he did far more than consult; he organized a team of scientists and began to screen thousands of soil samples in the search for a new antibiotic. Disappointment followed disappointment, but finally, in 1946, he found a golden mold that produced "something" having activity against about 50 different organisms that could cause disease. From this mold came chlortetracycline, the first of the broad-spectrum antibiotics. Lederle gave it the trade name, Aureomycin, a term derived from *aureus*, the Latin word for gold, and *Actinomycete*, the scientific name of the group of microorganisms from which it was isolated. The sample of soil from which the golden mold was grown had been scooped up on the campus of the University of Missouri, where Professor Duggar once was a member of the faculty.

The initial tests in which the new antibiotic was used to

treat diseased animals were not spectacular, and some scientists, both within and outside the Lederle organization, were pessimistic about its probable value in clinical medicine. Extensive testing in the clinic, however, requiring several years to complete, established its efficacy against a number of infectious diseases in humans. In addition to its effectiveness against the usual gram-positive and gram-negative organisms, it was found to have activity against a curious group of microorganisms known as rickettsia. These latter organisms cause Rocky Mountain spotted fever, typhus, and parrot fever in man. The new antibiotic was marketed by Lederle in 1949.

Aureomycin proved to be the first of a group of antibiotics now known as the tetracyclines. Another member of this group, oxytetracycline, was discovered in the research laboratories of Pfizer, and marketed in 1950 under its trademark, Terramycin. Tetracycline, another member of the series, is marketed by several other firms under various trade names, and other tetracycline derivatives are also available.

Dr. Duggar died in 1956, ten years after his discovery of Aureomycin—"the golden one."

CHAPTER 5

The FDA and New Drugs

A Bit of History. Recent Decline
in New Drugs. Some Philosophy

ALTHOUGH THERE ARE many significant dates in the history of food and drug law in the United States, three of them have special importance to the drug trade. In each case, several years of debate in the Congress preceded the passage of legislation; in each case, Congress was spurred to action by upsurges of public interest, generated by revelations that the American people believed demonstrated dramatic threats to public health. In each case, also, the President of the United States requested the Congress to take action.

Dr Harvey W. Wiley often has been referred to as the "father" of the original Pure Food and Drug Act, also known as the Heyburn Act. It passed Congress and was signed June 30, 1906, by President Theodore Roosevelt. On the same day the President signed a companion bill, the Meat Inspection Act. Dr. Wiley had an MD degree, but he also had studied chemistry at Harvard for two years, and undoubtedly considered himself a chemist. His early medical training may have led to his high interest in the flood of impure and spurious drugs that flowed into the US market prior to 1906. He made his first mark as state chemist of Indiana, became Chief of the Bureau of Chemistry of the Department of Agriculture on April 9, 1883, and from this position led the fight for the passage of a law that would regulate marketed foods and drugs. He published a classic bulletin, *Foods and Food Adulterants,* in the late 1880s. The first really encouraging sign of progress came in the 57th Congress, when the House passed a pure-food bill early in the second session. The Senate failed to act, however, before adjournment in March, 1903.

In 1903, the American Medical Association revived an old campaign against secret medicines and quack remedies. This stimulated Dr. Wiley to organize a drug laboratory to analyze such drugs, and he began to campaign against them. In 1904, *The Ladies' Home Journal* published a series of editorials, written by Edward Bok, which revealed that many popular remedies were worthless and that many of them contained relatively high concentrations of alcohol and habit-forming drugs. *The Journal* had banned the advertising of medicines from its pages twelve years earlier. During 1905 and 1906, a group of articles entitled "The Great American Fraud," also devoted to the exposure of fradulent drugs, was published in *Collier's* by Samuel Hopkins Adams. On February 1, 1906, the Senate passed a pure-food bill, but there was a disturbing delay in the House. The bill might have died there if it had not been for the publication of a novel, *The Jungle*, by Upton Sinclair. *The Jungle* contained gruesome descriptions of the careless handling of meat in the Chicago stockyards, and there was a public clamor for legislation. President Roosevelt told Speaker Cannon of the House that he wanted action, and on June 23 the House passed an even stronger bill than that passed by the Senate. Four days later, both houses accepted a compromise conference committee report. The President signed the bill on June 30, 1906.

The new law recognized as official two compendia that listed minimal standards for those drugs that the majority of the health professions believed useful in the treatment of disease. Although *The United States Pharmacopeia* (USP) had been in existence since 1820, and *The National Formulary* (NF) since 1888, no legal way of enforcing their standards had existed. It was the intent of the law to require that the label of a marketed drug must list all active ingredients truthfully, and give directions for use that were in accord with the results of the pharmacologic and clinical studies. A ruling of the Supreme Court in August, 1912, however, made it clear that the government did not have the power to rule on curative claims. In 1922, a federal judge ruled that "no law prohibits a man from making any medicine he wants to and selling it to the people if he tells the truth about it."

The enforcement of the new bill was entrusted to the Bureau of Chemistry of the Department of Agriculture, and Dr. Wiley, as Chief of the Bureau, set up an efficient enforcement machinery. It is noteworthy, too, that the bill had nothing to say about new drugs prior to marketing, but it did force manufacturers to establish quality-control procedures for marketed drugs. Today, many of the control procedures used for marketed drugs are developed in the research and development area of the pharmaceutical company as the drug is being studied prior to marketing.

Although no one can deny that Dr. Wiley was a dedicated and crusading scientist determined to do his best to insure that marketed drugs and foods were pure, unadulterated, and properly labeled, he did prove, nevertheless, that even the most conscientious of government enforcement agencies can make mistakes in judgment. Dr. Wiley became convinced that sodium benzoate, used in low concentrations as a preservative for foods and drugs, and saccharin, used as a sweetening agent, were toxic. He requested President Roosevelt to ban their use in foods and drugs. Dr. Wiley himself has stated that the President at first had decided to follow his advice about sodium benzoate, but reversed this decision when he learned of Dr. Wiley's position on saccharin. It seems that the President's own physician had prescribed saccharin for his use and from his own experience with the substance he thought it was safe. In fact, the President has been quoted as saying: "Anybody who says saccharin is injurious to health is an idiot."

As a result of Dr. Wiley's position, President Roosevelt appointed the so-called Remsen Board, composed of eminent scientists, to investigate the potential toxicity of sodium benzoate and saccharin. Their report gave to both a clear bill of health, and the President lost confidence in Dr. Wiley's judgment, and appointed a Board to administer the Bureau of Chemistry. A short time later, in 1921, Dr. Wiley left and joined the staff of *Good Housekeeping*. In 1927, a separate law-enforcement agency of the Department of Agriculture was created. Its first name was the Food, Drug, and Insecticide Administration, changed in 1931 to the Food and Drug Administration (FDA). Mr. Walter C. Campbell, formerly Chief of the Bureau of Chemistry, became the first Chief of the new Administration.

Only a few days after President Franklin D. Roosevelt was inaugurated, one of his new Assistant Secretaries of Agriculture, Rexford Tugwell, had a discussion with Mr. Campbell, Chief of the FDA, and both men agreed that the existing food and drug laws did not provide adequate safeguards for the consumer. That same day, the President authorized Mr. Tugwell to prepare a revision of the Pure Food and Drug Act for presentation to the Congress. As it turned out, this authorization marked the beginning of a five-year battle ending in the passage of the Federal Food, Drug, and Cosmetic Act in 1938.

As in 1906, passage of the new act was triggered by an episode that profoundly shocked the public, the Congress, and the President. During the period September 4 through October 15, 1938, a pharmaceutical house distributed 240 gallons of a drug labeled "Elixir of Sulfanilamide" for sale. It was a liquid solution of sulfanilamide in a flavored solvent composed of diethylene glycol and water. Prior to marketing, the pharmaceutical house had made no investigations of potential toxicity in animals or in humans. According to the Secretary of Agriculture's report, ninety three persons who took the medication died. They resided in fifteen states, as far east as Virginia and as far west as California. At least seventy three of them died as a direct result of taking the new drug. The twenty other victims had received multiple medications, but the suspicion was strong that the Elixir was the responsible agent. The toxicity was caused by the diethylene glycol, which had not previously been used as a solvent for drugs.

As a result of strenuous efforts by the government and by the pharmaceutical company, all of the distributed drug was accounted for, and all unused material was recovered. Diethylene glycol was not disclosed on the label, but, since it was not claimed as an active ingredient, this did not give legal grounds for seizure and removal of the product from the market. Instead, the government took the position that the drug was mislabeled because the term "Elixir" was used on the label. Technically, an elixir was defined as a drug in which the solvent used was a mixture of water and ethyl alcohol (ordinary grain alcohol). Chemically speaking, diethylene glycol was an alcohol but of course was not identical with ethyl alcohol.

The Food, Drug, and Cosmetic Act then pending in Congress did not contain governmental controls over new drugs prior to marketing. An aroused Congress quickly added a new Section 505 to deal with this problem. This section provided that a New Drug Application (NDA) must be submitted to the FDA prior to marketing a new drug in interstate commerce. Required information in the NDA included, among other things, a full report of investigations in animals and humans to show that the drug was safe for use; a full statement of the composition of the new drug; a full statement of the methods used in, and facilities and controls used for, the manufacturing, processing, and packaging of the drug; and specimens of the labeling proposed to be used. The law provided that the NDA should become effective on the sixtieth day after filing unless the Administrator of the FDA in writing postponed the effective date to such time (not to exceed 180 days after filing) as deemed necessary. In other words, the FDA was not required to make an affirmative ruling unless its staff decided that the new drug was too toxic to justify marketing, or unless some other provision of Section 505 was not satisfied. After the elapsed time specified by the bill, and in the absence of a negative FDA ruling, the manufacturer was free to market the drug.

The new law also included a definition of the term "new drug," which has caused considerable controversy between pharmaceutical manufacturers and the FDA whether certain drugs were, by this definition, "new drugs" or "old drugs." New drugs were defined as *a*) substances that had not been used sufficiently as drugs to become generally recognized as safe; *b*) combinations of well known drugs when such combinations had not become generally recognized as safe; and *c*) well known drugs and combinations of drugs bearing label directions for higher dosage or more frequent dosage or for longer duration of use than had become generally recognized as safe. The law required the FDA to issue regulations exempting from the operation of Section 505 drugs intended solely for investigational use by experts qualified by scientific training and experience to investigate the safety of drugs. In other words, the investigation of new drugs prior to submission of an NDA was entirely the responsibility of the manufacturer.

In actual practice, approval of an NDA often required months or even years longer than the statutory 180 days. The simplest reason was that the FDA scientific staff was woefully undermanned. The tremendous work load is underlined by the fact that more than 14,000 NDAs were received and processed between 1938 and 1965. It was quite customary, therefore, for the FDA to turn down an NDA, usually on day 60 to 180, on the grounds that the information contained therein was incomplete. Often it seemed to the pharmaceutical house that the additional information required was insignificant. The only practical recourse was to resubmit the amended NDA and to wait out the additional time (up to 180 days) thus gained by the FDA. It was possible to appeal a negative ruling of the FDA by filing in a district federal court, but this procedure generally was thought to involve even more delay than that needed to resubmit the amended NDA. Moreover, it hardly improved relations between the complaining company and the staff of the FDA. In some cases, also, the FDA seemingly took the position that a new drug that they believed to be ineffective, or even less effective than a marketed drug, was toxic. The reasoning was that the patient would be damaged by taking the less effective drug, since usually this meant that he would not receive the benefit that might have accrued had he been given that more effective.

On July 1, 1940, the Federal Security Agency was created, and the FDA was transferred from the Department of Agriculture to this Agency. The new Agency reported to President Roosevelt, but its head did not have Cabinet rank. On April 11, 1953, during President Eisenhower's administration, the Federal Security Agency became the United States Department of Health, Education and Welfare (HEW). The Secretary of the new department was a member of the Cabinet, and the FDA, as a part of it, was headed by an officer with the rank of Commissioner. In 1968, further changes were made in the organization of the HEW. The Commissioner of the FDA now reports to the Administrator of the Consumer Protection and Environmental Service. This Administrator reports to the Assistant Secretary for Health and Scientific Affairs, who, in turn, reports to the Secretary of HEW.

An important amendment to the Federal Food, Drug, and Cosmetic Act was enacted on October 26, 1951. Known as the Durham-Humphrey Amendment, it required that drugs that cannot be used safely without medical supervision be dispensed only on prescription, and also provided that a special type of label be used for packaging of the drug. The important features of this label were the inclusion of a statement that the drug was intended for prescription dispensing only and the omission of the medical indications for its use, since pertinent information needed by physicians and pharmacists was to be included in a circular accompanying each package of the drug.

Another important amendment was enacted on July 6, 1945. It required certification of the safety and efficacy of penicillin; that is, it required that no production batch of penicillin be marketed until it had been examined and approved by the FDA. Later amendments extended this requirement to other antibiotics, and the Kefauver-Harris Amendments of 1962 required certification for essentially all marketed antibiotics. The principle of certification was not initiated by the 1945 amendment. Since December 22, 1941, all production lots of insulin, by law, have been certified by the FDA prior to marketing.

The third date of special importance in the history of food and drug law is October 10, 1962. On this day President Kennedy signed into law the Kefauver-Harris Drug Amendments. The passage of this bill was marked by the disclosure of a therapeutic catastrophe that profoundly shocked the American public, the Congress, and the President. In fact, the President demanded drastic and immediate action by the Congress—and got it.

About three years earlier, Senator Estes Kefauver, as Chairman of the Subcommittee on Antitrust and Monopoly of the

Judiciary Committee of the Senate, had begun an investigation of the prices of drugs. During these lengthy sessions it became clear that the FDA believed it needed more power to regulate new drugs, both during the developmental stages and after marketing. Senator Kefauver agreed with this view and introduced a bill in the Senate early in 1961; a similar bill was introduced in the House by Representative Harris.

While these bills were being debated in committees of the Senate and the House, the public became aware of the tragic history of the drug, thalidomide. A German physician had called attention to the toxicity of the drug (marketed in Europe since 1957) at a medical meeting held on November 22, 1961. *Time* correspondents had sent a report of this meeting to Gilbert Cant, the magazine's medicine editor. He checked and, finding that the drug was not marketed in the United States, decided against publishing the story. Later he became aware that thalidomide (trademarked Contergan in Europe) was marketed under the trademark Kevadon in Canada and actually was on clinical trial in the United States. *Time* then carried the story in its issue of February 23, 1962. Meanwhile, the William S. Merrell Company, the United States firm that was studying the drug clinically with a view to marketing it in this country, undertook a thorough investigation of the situation, and as a result, withdrew its New Drug Application in March, 1962.

Thalidomide had been discovered in the laboratories of the German firm, Chemie Grünenthal. It displayed anticonvulsant activity in animal tests, and was investigated clinically as a potential agent of value in the treatment of epilepsy. It turned out to be ineffective in this disorder but surprisingly, proved an excellent sleep-inducing drug. (It had not caused sedation or sleepiness in animals.) Moreover, it appeared to be far safer than were the commonly used barbiturates, and by the end of 1957, it was widely used in Europe. In this country, the Merrell Company acquired the rights to market the drug, and undertook the necessary laboratory and clinical studies. During 1961, some cases of polyneuritis were reported in patients who had received the drug. Of far greater importance, however, was the finding that its use by pregnant women had been associated with the birth of several thousand babies who exhibited serious birth defects, the most common the condition known as phocomelia. In thèse babies, the hands—and sometimes the feet—seemed to be attached directly to the body without the intervention of a limb, and thus resembled the flippers of a seal. (The term *phocomelia* is derived from two Greek words meaning seal and extremity.) All of the reported cases had occurred abroad; none had been observed as a result of clinical trials of the drug in the United States.

The story published in *Time* apparently did not make too much impression on the public and on government officials in Washington. On July 15, however, a story about thalidomide and the tragic consequences following its use abroad was published in the *Washington Post*. This caused almost immediate reaction in the Congress and in the White House.

On August 1, 1962, President Kennedy called for the passage of a strong drug law, specifically asking that the bill before the Senate be strengthened to allow for immediate removal from the market of a drug when there was immediate hazard to public health. On August 23, the Senate passed, by unanimous vote, a much more extreme bill than the one that had been under consideration just prior to the publication of the thalidomide story in the *Washington Post*. The House did not react in so hysterical a fashion; indeed, the bill was almost killed. When the Rules Committee of the House first voted on whether or not to refer it to the floor, the vote was six for and six against. If this vote had been the final one, it would have meant that the bill was killed until a future session of the Congress. However, Congressman Harris, author of the bill, went before the Committee and explained that the Pharmaceutical Manufacturers Association supported the bill. A new vote was taken and the bill was passed by a vote of eight to four. The final bill, a compromise worked out by a joint committee of the Senate and the House, was passed by the Senate on October 3 and by the House on October 4. The President signed it into law on October 10.

The new amendments gave the FDA sweeping authority over new drugs extending from the time of proposed first clinical trials through production and marketing. It provided that each drug-manufacturing establishment be registered annually and be inspected at least once every two years by FDA inspectors. Drugs were defined as adulterated, and hence subject to seizure and removal from the market, if they had not been produced in a plant operated in conformity with good manufacturing practice. False or misleading labeling (including information on package inserts) was prohibited, both at the time of marketing and at any time thereafter, and information that must appear on labels was specified. Power to regulate the content of advertising for prescription drugs was given to the FDA; previously this had been a function of the Federal Trade Commission. The FDA was required to test and certify each production lot of an antibiotic intended for human use prior to marketing. Strict record keeping was required and such records were to be made available to FDA inspectors on request. When desirable, the FDA could designate a standard official name for a new drug.* The Secretary of the Department of

---

* In actual practice, usually the manufacturer submits suggested names to an organization known as the United States Adopted Name Council (USAN), formed January 2, 1964. The five members of this Council represent the American Medical Association, the US Pharmacopeial Convention, and the American Pharmaceutical Association. In 1967, the FDA agreed to supply an additional member. If all members of USAN agree on a name, it will be accepted by the FDA as the established or official name. If there is not unanimous agreement, the Commissioner of the FDA reserves the right to select a name.

HEW was required to furnish information about new drugs to the Commissioner of Patents when requested to do so, and was given the power to remove a drug from the market without a hearing if he believed that the drug was an immediate hazard to public health.

Of most concern to us are the amendments that apply specifically to studies of new drugs prior to marketing. Sponsors of new drug investigations in humans are required to submit preclinical tests adequate to justify that proposed investigation. They must obtain signed agreements from each clinical investigator that the new drug will be used only under his supervision, and are required to obtain the consent of the human subjects who are to participate in the investigation unless it is not feasible to do so, or, in their professional judgment, it is contrary to the best interests of the patient.

Of great importance is the amended definition of a new drug. To the definition just stated here (see page 84), the law added, to *a*), *b*), and *c*), *and effective*. In other words, new drugs cannot be marketed in interstate commerce until substantial evidence of both safety and effectiveness have been furnished to the FDA. There is no longer automatic approval to market in the absence of unfavorable FDA reaction; affirmative approval by the FDA to market is mandatory. The new law allows the FDA 180 days (or additional time if agreed to by the sponsor) for *initial* consideration of a New Drug Application. (In the event of disapproval by the FDA, the sponsor may request a hearing before the FDA. This procedure seldom has been used, probably because it seems unlikely that it would result in a reversal of the negative decision already voiced by the Agency.)

Detailed regulations implementing the new Amendments were issued by the FDA in 1963, and additional or amended regulations have appeared from time to time since then. These

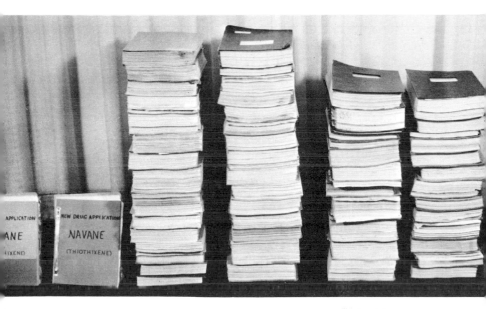

The complete NDA for thiothixene (Navane, J. B. Roerig Division of Chas. Pfizer & Company, Inc.) consisted of 46 volumes of some 46,000 pages. The two volumes at the left comprise the Summary. (PFIZER)

regulations specify the documents and procedures already described in Chapter 2, and require that the sponsor monitor each investigation of the new drug, evaluate it, and submit reports to the FDA at least once each year. Any findings suggesting that the new drug is hazardous must be reported immediately to the Agency and the investigations in progress be suspended until a decision may be reached that it is safe to continue. They provide that adequate records be kept for at least 2 years after the drug is marketed or after the investigations have been discontinued. They also describe various conditions under which the FDA can order termination of clinical investigations and require sponsors to recall unused supplies of the drug. These conditions are numerous, ranging all the way from the inclusion of untrue statements in the IND, inadequate manufacturing or control procedures, or substantial evidence to show that the drug is unsafe.

During the 11-year period, 1957-1968, and especially since 1962, the date of passage of the new Amendments, the average number of new drugs marketed annually, and particularly the number of new entities, has diminished appreciably. This statement is illustrated by the following table, assembled from data compiled by Paul De Haen of New York City.

YEAR	NUMBER OF FIRMS	TOTAL NEW PRODUCTS	NEW SINGLE CHEMICALS	DUPLICATE SINGLE PRODUCTS	COMBINATION PRODUCTS	NEW DOSAGE FORMS
1957	127	400	51	88	261	96
1958	126	370	44	73	253	109
1959	107	315	63	49	203	104
1960	109	306	45	62	199	98
1961	111	260	39	32	189	106
1962	108	250	27	43	180	84
1963	89	199	16	34	149	52
1964	82	157	17	29	111	41
1965	65	112	23	18	71	22
1966	52	80	12	15	53	26
1967	49	82	25	25	32	14
1968	48	87	11	26	50	21

12-yr total   2,618
New dosage forms   773
    Grand total   3,391

The table also indicates that the number of firms marketing new ethical products has declined steadily since 1962. The column headed *Total New Products* does not include new dosage forms, which really are not new drugs but rather pharmaceutical variations (tablets, capsules, liquids, suppositories, and so on) of drugs already marketed. Nevertheless, every new dosage form requires the submission of an NDA to establish safety and efficacy. Indeed, the marketing of every new drug, even duplicates of drugs already on the market, requires that the manufacturer submit his own data in support of an NDA. Of course one manufacturer may permit another manufacturer to refer to data previously filed with the FDA, but this is unusual except in cases where one firm licenses another to market an approved drug.

There are several reasons for the recent decline in the number of new ethical drugs marketed each year. One cause, strangely enough, is a tremendous increase in scientific knowledge and technology that are useful in the evaluation of drugs. Advances in analytic technics make it possible to detect inpurities in new chemical substances that would have been overlooked in the past. When such impurities are detected, further laboratory studies are initiated in the attempt to find methods of removing them. If, from a practical point of view, this cannot be accomplished, then accurate control procedures must be devised in order to insure that unusual amounts of the impurities do not appear in production batches of the new drug. Efforts to isolate and identify the impurities are made, since a knowledge of their chemical structures may provide clues to their potential effects on toxicity and efficacy of the drug, and procedures for the control of the levels of impurities are required prior to the initiation of long-term toxicity studies, since, obviously, variations in these levels may influence the results of such studies.

Biochemical studies designed to give as much information as possible about the fate of the drug in the animal body are usually carried out. In many cases in the past, this type of investigation was not done because the technics available were inadequate. These studies indicate the organs in which the new drug tends to concentrate after absorption, the length of time it remains in the body, whether it is altered chemically in the body and, if so, the number of metabolites (new products formed in the tissues from the drug) formed and excreted. In some cases, it is possible even to identify these metabolites.

It is becoming increasingly evident that biochemical studies may help greatly in devising suitable toxicity studies; for example, suppose that a new drug is metabolized in the rat in such fashion that four metabolites are excreted in the urine. Perhaps this same drug, when given to dogs, is excreted as only two metabolites, possibly but not necessarily identical with two of the metabolites in the urine of the rats. If the first trials of the new agent in the human indicate that he handles the drug metabolically like the rat (that is, he excretes the same four metabolites as the rats), then it is highly probable that toxicity studies done in the rat will be much more meaningful than similar studies done in the dog. This is true because it is possible that some of the toxicity exhibited by the drug may be due to one or more of the metabolites rather than to the drug itself.

Methods of detecting toxicity have become more subtle and sophisticated. Injury to some organs results in the release of enzymes into the blood; the chemical detection of these enzymes can indicate toxicity even though there is no external indication of it. Histologic technics have improved tremendously also; tissues taken from the bodies of animals sacrificed in toxicity studies can be examined with the ultramiscroscope, and changes that cannot be seen with the ordinary microscope detected. New staining methods make it possible to evaluate the ability of cells to carry out essential or desirable chemical reactions. It is even possible now to separate cells into various subcellular particles, which then can be examined by technics that make it possible to judge whether these particles are normal, both anatomically and functionally. Individual cells can be grown in tissue culture, and the effect of the new drug on them in the test tube can be studied. When these newer procedures indicate possible toxicity, more careful and more lengthy studies usually are carried out today than in former years.

Prior to 1962, when the tragic story of thalidomide became known, it had not been customary to test new drugs in pregnant animals or to do toxicity studies in newborn animals. Indeed, it required many investigations carried out all over the world to discover a test procedure that could detect the teratogenic potential (power to produce deformities in the unborn) of thalidomide itself. A procedure, in which rabbits of a specific type (New Zealand white rabbits) were used as test animals, was worked out in an English laboratory, and now is used generally in preclinical studies of new drugs. Another successful procedure, much more time-consuming, involves the use of monkeys as test animals. It is interesting, and somewhat disconcerting, to find that many older drugs, including even aspirin, exhibit some degree of teratogenicity when they are subjected to the tests now generally used to detect such activity in potential new drugs. Because these older drugs have not caused apparent difficulty of this type in the human, it is obvious that the present test procedures are far from perfect. However, I believe that nearly all, if not all, scientists concerned with the development of new drugs believe that they should not be administered to women of child-bearing age (or more properly to women capable of bearing children, since some women of child-bearing age are known to be sterile) until the presently available animal tests are performed and evaluated.

If a fool-proof way of insuring that women able to bear children did not ingest the drug, thalidomide probably would be a highly useful therapeutic agent. It has the great advantage over the barbiturates that it is almost nontoxic, except for its teratogenic properties. It is almost impossible to give enough of it to animals to cause death or, even, signs of toxicity. In the human, unlike the barbiturates, it has no effect on respiration or on the action of the heart. This practically eliminates the possibility of accidental death or suicide through its use. One person is known to have attempted to commit suicide by ingesting 144 times the usual dose, but he survived. In some areas of the world, thalidomide still is used in hospitals. The cases in which peripheral neuritis was associated with the administration of thalidomide occurred after administration of the drug for a long time. In any case, they were too few in number to prove conclusively that the drug was the cause of the neuritis.

Advances in the methodology involved in testing new drugs in humans also have contributed to the increase in the time required to evaluate a new drug. Ten years ago, it was quite customary to supply a potential new drug to clinicians who were experts in the management of the condition for which the new agent was intended; the opinions of these experts served to "make or break" the new drug. Today, clinical trials are done on a much more objective basis: they are planned carefully with the aid of statisticians so that results can be evaluated objectively. Moreover, many of the trials are controlled—that is, the new agent is compared with a placebo (inactive material such as milk sugar) or with one or more established drugs in such a way that the patients (and, ideally, the physicians supervising the study of the test drug) do not know which test material they have received. Much more elaborate tests of potential toxicity, involving sensitive laboratory procedures only recently available, also are done today. More sensitive and objective measurements that indicate utility, or lack of it, have been devised in recent years, which increase greatly our confidence that new drugs are safe and effective, although the time required for evaluation has increased greatly.

Another reason for the slowdown in the discovery of new drugs is simply that we have exhausted much of the fundamental biologic knowledge required to develop meaningful laboratory tests of potential clinical utility. If we use the same old tests available in the past, it is not surprising that new drugs often are only variations of older drugs. That is why it is so important for the biologists in the pharmaceutical industry to devote a sizeable portion of their efforts to the accumulation of new scientific knowledge.

An important reason for the decline in the emergence of new drugs is, in my opinion, the judgments made by the staff of the FDA. Prior to the submission of an NDA to the FDA, the pharmaceutical company has spent, quite literally, millions of dollars in developing the potential new drug to this final stage. The capable, highly trained scientists of the pharmaceutical company have evaluated the information available and have concluded that it is sufficient to justify marketing the new agent. In view of the tremendous investment involved, it just does not make sense that they would make this judgment capriciously. And yet the scientists in the FDA more often than not disagree with their peers in the industry. Dr. James L. Goddard, then Commissioner of the FDA, quoted some revealing figures in testimony given to the Monopoly Subcommittee of the Senate Select Small Business Committee on August 10, 1967. He stated that five times as many NDAs were found to be not approvable (as judged by the staff of the FDA) as were approved. Obviously, in Dr. Goddard's opinion, this situation was not caused by the conservatism of the staff of the FDA, but was the fault of the scientists in the Industry. Indeed, he said: "There is no reason why a manufacturer cannot do the job properly the first time." He conceded that the Industry has challenged evalutions made by the FDA, but added: "This is our evaluation, and I am prepared to stand by it."

Now if a disagreement about adequacy of data exists between the industrial scientists and the FDA staff, the FDA holds all the aces, and, in practice, always can win the argument. True enough, the Amendments of 1962 provide that if a pending NDA is disapproved, a hearing can be requested by the manufacturer. "If the applicant elects to accept the opportunity for hearing by written request within thirty days after such notice, such hearing shall commence not more than ninety days after the expiration of such thirty days unless the Secretary"—of HEW—"and the applicant otherwise agree. Any such hearing shall thereafter be conducted on an expedited basis and the Secretary's order thereon shall be issued within ninety days after the date fixed by the Secretary for filing final briefs." It is apparent that this procedure involves a long period of time, with not much chance of a reversal of the FDA's decision (the hearing is before the parent organization of the FDA). If, after a hearing, the decision still is unfavorable to the manufacturer, the issue can be taken to the federal courts, but final resolution of the controversy by this procedure usually would require very long periods of time, years rather than months. In most cases, then, when an NDA is not approved, the scientific and clinical staffs of the applicant undertake the additional investigations thought to be necessary by the FDA. All too often when the revised NDA, now including the new information, is submitted, the FDA decides that, in its judgment, still more data are required, and so the already lengthy process is repeated.

Why are the judgments made by the FDA so much more conservative than those made by the Industry? For the last ten years, the activities of the FDA have been under almost constant investigation by various Subcommittees of the Congress. In those few instances where new drugs have been withdrawn from the market because of excessive toxicity, the Congress and the public have been inclined to blame the FDA for its decision to allow marketing. I believe all this has created an unduly cautious attitude on the part of the FDA scientist. If he makes a mistake in approving the marketing of a new drug, he and the Agency are blamed. If he does not grant approval, only the manufacturer is unhappy. In other words, it is psychologically much easier for the FDA to say *no* than to say *yes*.

This raises an important question. How many lives have been lost in the recent past, or will be lost in the future, because the marketing of live-saving drugs has been delayed by judgments that are too conservative? Perhaps this question can be answered ten years from now. It is at least possible that in an overall sense the health of the public is no better protected today than it was prior to October, 1962.

In the period 1940 through 1967, 857 major new drugs were made available to the American physician. Only a handful of these have been removed from the market because of toxicity. When removal has occurred, in most cases the toxicity was observed only after the drug had been used for a considerable length of time in actual clinical practice, so that literally millions of patients had received it. This is not, in my opinion, a bad record. It will be most interesting, in retrospect, to learn whether the record of the next quarter of a century is better.

CHAPTER 6

Biologics

Some History—and Definitions, Properties.
Licensing and Enforcement. Development.
Number of Recent Products.

THE GROUP OF DRUGS known as biological products, biologicals, or biologics has no scientific definition. There is a legal one, however: Biologics are drugs that can be marketed only if they are manufactured in licensed establishments and if they are licensed by the Division of Biologics Standards, DBS (or, more accurately, by its parent organization, the Department of Health, Education, and Welfare, HEW). The DBS is a division of the National Institutes of Health, NIH. Until recently, the Director of the NIH reported to the Surgeon General of the Public Health Service, who, in turn, reported to the Secretary of the HEW. In 1968, the HEW was reorganized, and the Director of the NIH and the Surgeon General of the Public Health Service now report separately to the Assistant Secretary for Health and Scientific Affairs. The Assistant Secretary reports directly to the Secretary of the HEW.

Section 351 of the Public Health Service Act states that a biological product is "any virus, therapeutic serum, toxin, antitoxin, or analagous product, or arsphenamine or its derivates (or any other trivalent organic arsenic compound) applicable to the prevention, treatment, or cure of diseases or injuries of man." Since this statement mentions the first real chemotherapeutic agent (arsphenamine), it might be supposed that the intent of the authors of the bill was to include this type of drug in the definition. However, modern chemotherapeutic agents,

100

such as the sulfa drugs and antibiotics, are not regarded as biologics, and are not licensed by the DBS. Modern drugs defined as biologics are all of them vaccines, antitoxins, therapeutic serums, allergenic products, human blood intended for transfusion, and products prepared from human blood. Of course products not shipped in interstate commerce (such as blood collected for use in local hospitals) are not included.

There are approximately 300 different biologics licensed for sale in the United States. Some examples are:

Measles vaccines
Poliomyelitis vaccines
Pertussis (whooping cough) vaccines
Smallpox vaccines
Rabies vaccines
Immune serum globulin (human)
Citrated whole blood (human)
Diphtheria toxoid
Tetanus toxoid

The term *biologic* apparently originated spontaneously in the government, the industry, or both. Like the term *ethical drug*, it has no recognized birthday. Most dictionaries do not include the word as a noun. However, *Webster's Third New International Dictionary, Unabridged* gives this definition: "Biologic or biological: a biological product (such as a globulin, serum, vaccine, antitoxin, or antigen) used in the prevention or treatment of disease." And *The Random House Dictionary of The English Language* gives this: "—*n.* 3. *Pharm.* a biochemical product, as a serum, vaccine, antitoxin, or antigen, used in the diagnosis, prevention, or treatment of disease."

The events that led to the creation of the DBS began in the last century. The ancestor organization of the present Department of the Treasury of the Federal government was charged with the responsibility of collecting customs duties at ports of entry. Out of this function came a need for hospital facilities to care for sailors of the Merchant Marine (of the United States and other nations) and the Revenue Cutter Service (now the Coast Guard). The first such hospital was established in Norfolk, Virginia, in 1798, and as time went on, more hospitals sprang up in seaports and at ports such as those of the Great Lakes. These medical facilities were administered and staffed by the Marine Hospital Service, later to become the Public Health Service. One of the establishments within the Marine Hospital Service was the Hygienic Laboratory, an important function of which was to detect and identify diseases (and the microorganisms responsible for them) that might be brought into the United States by the sailors of the merchant ships. Some of these diseases, though uncommon in this country, were highly contagious and were obvious threats to the public health.

One of the first scientists in the United States to prepare and standardize diphtheria antitoxin was Dr. Joseph J. Kinyoun, of the Hygienic Laboratory. He was convinced that this, at that time, new type of drug required special care in its preparation and in the control of its potency, quality, and safety. In the early 1890s, he went to Paris and Berlin, where he learned about the experiences of European scientists who were investigating the preparation of antitoxins. In November, 1894, he wrote a report to Dr. Walter W. Wyman, Surgeon General of the Marine Hospital Service. One of its statements was:

> Many persons will, during the ensuing year, commence to prepare the serum as a business enterprise, and there will, without doubt, be many worthless articles called antitoxin thrown on the market. All the serum intended for sale should be made or tested by competent persons.

The testing, in fact, should be done by disinterested parties. . . .

In spite of the efforts of Dr. Kinyoun and others, Congress did not act until 1902. It was spurred to action (as when important food and drug laws were enacted) by a medical disaster that shocked the American people. Beginning in 1894, the City of St. Louis employed a bacteriologist to prepare diphtheria antitoxin from the blood of immunized horses, and to distribute it free to physicians. During 1901, a number of children who had received the diphtheria antitoxin died of tetanus (lockjaw). Investigation established that the blood of one of the horses used in the manufacture of the antitoxin contained live tetanus organisms, and was, then, the source of the infection.

The revelation of these deaths resulted in the introduction in Congress of legislation to control biological products. It was supported by the District of Columbia Medical Society and the DC authorities, and was handled in the Congress by the DC Committees of both Houses. Two important bills were enacted on July 1, 1902. One of these established the Public Health and Marine Hospital Service, thus providing for the first time an agency of the federal government that could coordinate public health affairs. The second Act authorized the new Service to regulate the sale and transportation for human use of viruses, serums, vaccines, antitoxins, and analogous products in interstate commerce or from any foreign country. This latter Act often is referred to as the "Virus-Toxin Law of 1902" or as the "Biologics Control Act."

Only three biological products existed in 1902: diphtheria antitoxin, tetanus antitoxin, and smallpox vaccine. The technical responsibility for control of these and future biologics was assigned to the Hygienic Laboratory, which previously had been the principal research and diagnostic group of the

Marine Hospital Service. When the Hygienic Laboratory was reorganized and expanded in 1930, its name was changed to the National Institute of Health. A Laboratory of Biologics Control was created within this Institute in 1937. Prior to its creation, the control of biologics was supervised by the Director of the National Institute of Health and, before him, by the Head of the Hygienic Laboratory. The Public Health Service was transferred from the Department of the Treasury to the newly established Federal Security Agency in 1940. In 1948, the old National Institute of Health was expanded organizationally to form the National Institutes of Health (NIH). The Laboratory of Biologics Control coincidentally became a part of the newly created National Microbiological Institute.

The Federal Security Agency was upgraded to the present Department of HEW on April 11, 1953, during President Eisenhower's administration. In June, 1955, the Secretary of HEW granted the Surgeon General of the PHS authority to expand the biologic control function by the creation of a separate division within the NIH to be named the Division of Biologics Standards (DBS). It was charged with the control of biologics and with the task of conducting a program of research related to the needs of adequate control. The DBS is responsible for establishing and maintaining standards of quality, safety, and potency of biologic products distributed in interstate commerce or from foreign countries.

Most biologics differ from other drugs in significant ways. Many of them are derived from living microorganisms, and are thus potentially infectious or potentially ineffective if improperly prepared and tested. Hence close surveillance of production and continuing programs to improve quality and testing procedures are necessary. The staff of the DBS includes competent scientists who are dedicated to the principle that the control of biologics requires a strong research base. Many biologics are used for the prevention or treatment of *acute* diseases and ordinarily only a few doses are used for any one recipient. Most commonly they are administered by injection. In the case of vaccines, usually one to three injections of the drug spread out over a period of weeks or months are given; booster (reinforcing) doses can then be given at intervals of a year or more, or following possible exposure to infection. Frequently, too, unlike most other drugs, many biologics are administered to persons in good health.

Most biologics obviously cannot be standardized by chemical or physical means. Hence their potency must be tested in animals or other biologic systems in comparison with an established standard preparation. The DBS provides standard preparations to manufacturers and others interested in biologics standardization. The development of these standards is a complex affair, and depends on knowledge in several fields of biologic science—for example, immunology, virology, bacteriology, biochemistry, and medicine. An acceptable standard must be stable under practical conditions of storage; it must yield sharp endpoints in the control testing carried out by all manufacturers and the DBS; and, desirably, gives results that correlate with those given by international standards or by standards established in other countries. A number of biologics standards have been adopted by the World Health Organization (WHO) and are official in most affiliated countries; usually the standard first developed for a new biologic is adopted by the WHO. Since many new biologics have been developed first in the United States, the DBS has a special responsibility to develop adequate and usable standards.

Biologics inherently are less stable than most other drugs. Usually they must be stored under refrigeration (36° to 44° Fahrenheit or 2° to 8° Centigrade); a few of them must be kept at a much lower temperature. For example, yellow fever vaccine should be stored at –70° Centigrade or 126° below freezing on the Fahrenheit scale. Biologics must, by law, "meet standards, designed to insure the continued safety, purity, and potency of such products, prescribed in regulations . . . " Since these drugs are not pure chemical compounds, the words *safety, purity, potency,* and *standards* have somewhat special meanings.

The *safety* of a biologic cannot be assured in an absolute sense. It can be defined as a *relative* freedom from harmful effect to the recipient, provided the drug is given prudently, and provided the character of the product and the condition of the recipient have been considered. As an example, influenza vaccine is made from virus grown in chick embryos; hence, influenza vaccine should be administered cautiously, or not at all, to individuals known to be sensitive to eggs, chicken, or chicken feathers.

A biologic is never *pure* in a chemical sense, since almost always it consists of a mixture of many substances. This type of product is considered *pure* if it is free of extraneous material, whether or not this material is in itself harmful. A pure product, for example, will be free of materials (pyrogens) that cause chills and fever in the recipient.

Potency is defined in a biologic sense. A potent biologic will cause a given biologic result as indicated by laboratory tests or by carefully controlled clinical data obtained by giving the product in the intended manner. In other words, the product must perform as claimed. Usually it is possible to determine performance; administration of the biologic causes a measurable effect in the recipient as determined in the clinic or in the laboratory.

Standards refers to procedures and specifications that apply to the manufacture and release for sale of biologics. They are prescribed in regulations issued by the Secretary of HEW, and are designed, of course, to insure the safety, purity, and potency of biologics. The word *standard* is used also to refer to a standard preparation that can be used as a means of calibrating potency or, in some cases, safety and purity.

Licensing is the instrument provided in the Public Health Service Act for the control of biologics. Revocation of a license is a severe penalty. If the license revoked covers a product, it must be removed from the market; if the license covering the manufacturing establishment is revoked, the manufacturer can no longer manufacture and sell any biologic. Two types of license, then, are granted. When a manufacturer requests a license for his manufacturing facility, he must be prepared to produce at least one product. In other words, an "establishment license" never is issued alone; a "product license" must be issued simultaneously. However, although each product requires a separate license, the manufacturing establishment is covered by a single license.

When application for a license is made, the manufacturer must give a complete description of his facilities, personnel, and the procedures involved in producing the product. Evidence of stability of the product and of clinical acceptability must be furnished. Samples of the finished product are sent to the DBS along with summaries of the results of tests designed to measure quality, purity, and potency. Often the DBS requires that several batches of the product be used in supplying this information in order to demonstrate consistency of production. The stability of the product must be studied, and indeed, often the staff of the DBS will check all of the proposed test procedures against the product. Proposed package literature and labels must be submitted. Members of the staff of the DBS inspect the manufacturing plant. If all required standards are met, the DBS recommends, through the office of the Director of the NIH, that a license be issued, through the office of the Secretary of HEW.

A licensed establishment is inspected by the DBS at least once a year, and samples and test reports of each manufactured lot of each licensed product must be submitted to the Division. All of the test reports are checked carefully, and often some of the submitted samples are tested in the DBS laboratories. The manufactured lot cannot be distributed until the manufacturer receives authorization from the DBS. (In a few cases, exceptions to this procedure have been granted for long-established products.)

Section 351 of the Public Health Service Act applies only to *licensed* biologics; in other words, it does not apply to products under laboratory or clinical investigation prior to licensing. In spite of this, in actual practice manufacturers of biologics and the staff of the DBS work closely together during the development of new biologics. It is advantageous to both groups to do so, and certainly benefits the public by avoiding unnecessary delay in the availability of a useful, sometimes life-saving drug. When an application for license is received, the DBS must issue standards. It cannot do so unless—or until—it has confirmed and approved the various testing procedures proposed by the manufacturer. In turn, unless the manufacturer knows the standards that will be issued, it is difficult for him to produce several lots that will meet the standards finally issued. In most cases, these difficulties have been overcome in a highly satisfactory manner throughout the years by close cooperation, sometimes almost collaboration, between the scientific staffs of the producer and the DBS.

The regulations governing the conduct of clinical investigations of new drugs issued by the FDA apply also to biologics. The FDA, however, has delegated the responsibility for monitoring and evaluating these investigations to the DBS. The usual IND form for a proposed biologic product must be submitted prior to beginning clinical trials, but it is sent directly to the DBS rather than to the FDA. In the case of biologics, the signal for marketing is not the approval of an NDA by the FDA, but rather is the issuance of a license by the Secretary of HEW.

Even after a new biologic is licensed and marketed, its control continues to be the responsibility of the DBS. Section 130.2 of the FDA New Drug Regulations specifically exempts products licensed under the Public Health Service Act from the provisions of the Foods and Drugs Laws governing new drugs. When difficulties with marketed biologics have arisen, Dr. Roderick Murray, Director of the DBS, and his capable staff have maintained the attitude that solving the manufacturing or testing problems by scientific investigation is preferable to precipitate revocation of licenses.

It is interesting that the first report of the Surgeon General of the PHS, dated June 17, 1904, listed 12 licensed products. Ten of them were produced in the United States, one in Germany and one in France. (When biologics sold in this country are made in other countries, the manufacturing establishments and individual products must be licensed.) By contrast, as of July 1, 1965, 212 manufacturing facilities were licensed and 1,308 product licenses (actually covering 291 basic products) were in effect.

The development of a biologic is a complicated, time-consuming procedure. For a virus vaccine, for example, the virus must be isolated from an infected human. Usually it must be grown in various types of cells maintained in tissue culture in order to work out a procedure for obtaining large quantities of the infectious agent. If the virus present in the vaccine is to be live, it must be attenuated in some way so that only minor

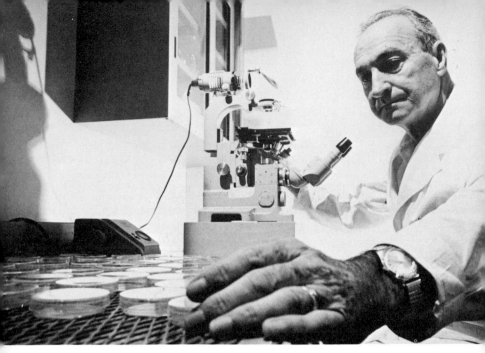

To make sure that unwanted viruses and contaminants do not get into the virus culture, many quality control checks are conducted. At MS&D, the vaccine is also quarantined a production batch at a time, until safety evaluations are confirmed by the Division of Biologics Standards. (MS&D)

signs of infection will be observed in subjects receiving it. (Live virus vaccines are believed to confer longer lasting protection than killed virus vaccines.) Quite literally, many thousands of animals, and probably at least 10,000 human subjects, must be used to obtain sufficient data to justify licensing.

To develop a live measles virus vaccine studied in the Merck Sharp & Dohme Research Laboratories, a virus strain isolated originally by Dr. J. F. Enders (a Nobel prize winner) and his associates at Harvard University was used. It was attenuated by being passed (grown) 24 times in primary cell cultures of human kidney, 28 times in primary human-amnion cell cultures, 12 times in embryonated hen's eggs, and 19 times in cell

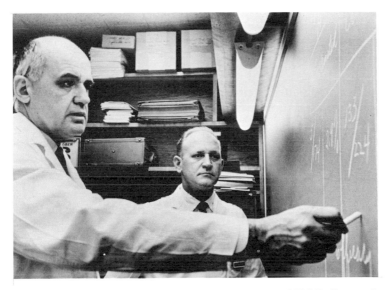

Developers of the live mumps virus vaccine at MS&D Research Laboratories, Drs. Hilleman and Buynak. Known as the Jeryl Lynn strain, the vaccine was derived from a virus isolated from Dr. Hilleman's daughter when she had mumps. (MS&D)

cultures of chick embryos. In the case of a live virus vaccine, exhaustive tests of safety are essential before the material is injected into humans. The Merck scientists tested their vaccine for safety in a variety of human and animal cell cultures (cellular damage indicates probable toxicity), in monkeys, mice, baby chicks, embryonated hen's eggs, and in a number of microbial culture media (to insure the absence of bacteria and other microorganisms other than viruses).

Licensed measles vaccines have been on the market since 1963. Early in 1968, Merck Sharp & Dohme marketed a new live virus mumps vaccine. Dr. Maurice R. Hilleman, Director of the Division of Virus and Tissue Culture Research of the Merck Institute for Therapeutic Research, really did his homework on this research project. The virus used in the development of the new vaccine was isolated from his five year old daughter, Jeryl Lynn, and has been named the Jeryl Lynn strain. The number of biologics licensed during the years 1960 through 1968 is given in the following table, compiled by Paul de Haen, well-known New York pharmaceutical consultant.

YEAR	TOTAL NEW PRODUCTS	NEW SINGLE BIOLOGIC ENTITIES	DUPLICATE BIOLOGIC ENTITIES	COMBINATION PRODUCTS
1960	5	0	2	3
1961	5	2	1	2
1962	5	1	4	0
1963	14	2	9	3
1964	5	0	5	0
1965	7	0	5	2
1966	2	1	1	0
1967	1	0	1	0
1968	14	3	10	1

CHAPTER 7

Animals and New Drugs

Essentials for Drug Research Ethics.
Regulation of Dealers. Laboratory
Care. Use in Screens

Would it be possible today to discover and develop new drugs without animal experimentation? No. I am sure that no clinical investigator would, on ethical grounds, give a potential new drug to humans if it had not first been studied in animals. Even if ethics were not involved, doing so would be illegal. The regulations implementing the Kefauver-Harris Drug Amendments of 1962 require that adequate animal experimentation, as outlined in Chapter 2, be performed and described in the document (IND) submitted to the FDA prior to clinical trial.

Even making the obviously false assumption that ethical and legal barriers do not exist, there would not be an adequate supply of human volunteers to permit the necessary screening, biologic and toxicity tests—nor would there be enough clinical investigators to do the job. The Pharmaceutical Manufacturers Association reported that its member firms (who account for about 95 percent of the new ethical drugs marketed in the United States) in 1968 used nearly 6.3 million mice; 2.4 million rats; 1,075,000 chickens; 129,000 guinea pigs; 78,000 rabbits; 39,000 dogs; 18,000 cats; and thousands of other birds and animals.

Observe that the great majority of these animals were mice and rats. The strains used in the search for new drugs have been developed by careful inbreeding for many generations.

Ideally, every male mouse, for example, should react exactly like every other male mouse when a new compound is given to him. In actual practice, however, in spite of the careful inbreeding, individual animals differ in their reactions to experimental procedures. In an actual acute toxicity test of a new compound, for example, the following results were obtained:

DOSE PER MOUSE	NUMBER OF MICE DYING	NUMBER OF MICE SURVIVING
60 mg	9	1
40 mg	6	4
30 mg	1	9
20 mg	0	10

Using mathematical calculations, these data indicate that a dose of 37.5 mg of the compound would be expected to kill one half of a large number of mice ingesting the drug. The mice used in this experiment, although highly inbred and of the same age, sex, and body weight, did differ in susceptibility to the new compound. Only one mouse survived a dose of 60 mg; only one died at a dose of 30 mg. Obviously human subjects would not be as closely related biologically as these mice were. It follows that huge numbers of humans would be required to obtain meaningful screening, biologic and toxicity information about potential new drugs.

It is true, of course that most of the drugs used during the first quarter of this century had been discovered without animal experimentation. Only a few of these drugs are used today. Among them are opium and its derivatives, quinine, atropine, iron salts, and aspirin; several laxatives—Epsom salt, castor oil, magnesium citrate, milk of magnesia, phenolphthalein, to mention a few—have also survived.

When I was a young pharmacist in Florida, the treatment of almost every illness included giving a laxative "to flush out

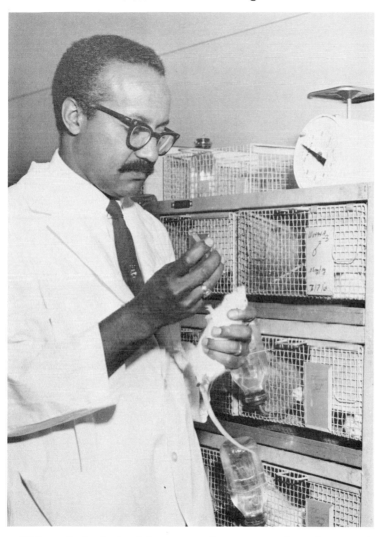

This toxicologist is giving a new drug to a rat in order to estimate its toxicity. (W-LRI)

poisons from the system." Often the drug used was calomel (mercurous chloride), followed by a dose of Epsom salt (magnesium sulfate) to "wash out the calomel." Many a child learned to dislike root beer because it was a favorite vehicle for castor oil. Children often were given sulfur and molasses in the spring; and people brewed a bitter tea ("tonic") from camomile. Although the practice was not condoned by physicians, some ignorant people tied smelly asafetida around their necks. Presumably they thought no disease germs would pass the odoriferous barrier thus created. This pitifully short list of useful older drugs is the heritage of thousands of years of human existence. By way of contrast, more than 800 new therapeutic entities have been made available in the United States since 1940. They were discovered and developed with the aid of animal experimentation.

What are the ethical considerations involved in our relationships with animals other than man? There is no single answer to this question. Each of us must, consciously or unconsciously, answer it in terms of some value system we regard as self-evident, that is, not subject to debate. Perhaps the principle stated by the late eminent biologist, Dr. A. J. Carlson of the University of Chicago, comes close to expressing the view of the majority of people in the United States. He wrote, "As between man and animals, man comes first."

Most of us have no compunction about injuring or killing the lower forms of animal life, for example, insects and worms. I believe there is a tendency to suppose that such forms of life really do not suffer pain as humans do. When the animal is a vertebrate—that is, has a brain, spinal cord, and backbone—most of us believe that pain and discomfort do enter the picture. Still, there is no widespread objection to catching fish with sharp hooks, and allowing them to die of asphyxiation when they are removed from water. Shooting birds and animals also is a popular sport. In some locations, and at certain times of the year, it is permissible, and apparently thought desirable, to hunt deer with bows and arrows, even though this method of hunting increases the chances of nonlethal injury with its accompanying pain and discomfort. For most people, of course, fishing and hunting are *sports;* it no longer is necessary to obtain food by these activities. With the possible exception of some vegetarians, people in this country do not object to the breeding and rearing of animals as sources of food, and of course we obtain leather and wool from animals also. I have talked to people who violently opposed animal experimentation but who saw nothing wrong or incongruous in wearing coats made from the skins of animals or feathers plucked from living birds. Branding unanesthetized cattle with hot irons also is acceptable to most people.

On the other hand, there are some people who oppose, in part or in whole, the use of living animals in scientific investigations, or in the training of students, scientists, and physicians. These people often are called antivivisectionists. The term *vivisection* is derived from Latin words meaning "to cut or section during life." Actually, only a small minority of the animal experiments carried out in the search for new drugs involves cutting procedures done on living animals. The figure probably approximates 5 percent. When operations must be performed, the animals are anesthetized. In many cases they are killed while still under anesthesia. If they are allowed to awaken, they are given careful postoperative care. This is not done on ethical grounds alone; to neglect the operated animals very likely would negate the experiment that required the operation. With the passage of time the word *vivisection* has acquired a broader meaning. *Webster's Third New International Dictionary, Unabridged,* includes the following definition: "broadly: any form of animal experimentation especially if considered to cause distress to the subject." Antivivisectionists, then, are people who oppose some or all animal experimentation.

Apparently, some antivivisectionists believe it is unethical for man to sacrifice the comfort or lives of animals for the purpose of scientific study under any conditions. *The New York Times Magazine* quotes Owen B. Hunt, president of the American Antivivisection Society, as stating bluntly: "Antivivisectionists oppose all experiments on animals even in trying to find a cure for other animals." Other people think that it is no less objectionable on ethical grounds to subject humans, rather than animals, to experimentation involving pain or discomfort. Major C. W. Hume, Secretary-General of the Universities Federation for Animal Welfare of Great Britain, in an article entitled "How to Befriend Laboratory Animals," has written:

> But when it comes to hurting, as distinct from killing, is there any reason why hurting an animal should be less objectionable than hurting a man with the same intensity? We must not allow this issue to be confused by the side issue of social repercussions. If you hurt a man, you also cause distress to his relatives and friends and you may incapacitate him from carrying out his social duties; these considerations do not arise in the case of an animal and they have to be taken into account, but they are irrelevant to the principle of our question and must not be allowed to confuse it. Apart from these social repercussions, is it more objectionable to hurt a man than an animal? I should say definitely not, and if anybody thinks that it is, it is pertinent to put the question "Why?"
>
> I know of no reason except prejudice for preferring that an animal rather than a random human being should suffer a given amount of pain, provided always that individual suffering be distinguished from its social repercussions and from the risk of death.

I believe it is fair to state that antivivisectionists as a group have a bias for the interests of animals as against the interests of fellow humans. Moreover, many of them obviously distrust scientists, and some even seem to regard them as sadists who enjoy torturing animals. On the contrary, scientists are *people*, and many of them have chosen to be biologists primarily because of their enjoyment of and love for animals. Many of them have pets at home.

A number of bills favored by antivivisectionists that have been introduced in Congress over the years have provided that bureaucrats in Washington, rather than trained biological or medical scientists, should decide whether proposed animal experimentation is permissible. One bill presented to (but not passed by) the 87th Congress specified that a Commissioner of Laboratory Animal Control be appointed by the President. He would have the power to approve or disapprove experiments involving living animals. What were his qualifications for making these complicated and important decisions? I quote from the bill:

> To be eligible for appointment as Commissioner, a candidate must have been admitted to practice law in the Supreme Court of the United States. No person who is or has ever been connected with any laboratory shall be eligible for appointment as Commissioner.

To me this seems quite as illogical as the suggestion that a highly qualified biologist be given the legal responsibility for defending a person accused of first degree murder.

In 1909, Dr. John Dewey, Professor of Philosophy at Columbia University, wrote an essay on "The Ethics of Animal Experimentation." In part, he wrote:

> What is the duty of the community regarding legislation that imposes *special* restrictions upon the persons engaged in scientific experimentation with animals? That

it is the duty of the state to pass *general* laws against cruelty to animals is a fact recognized by well nigh all civilized states. But opponents of animal experimentation are not content with such general legislation; they demand what is in effect—if not legally—class legislation, putting scientific men under peculiar surveillance and limitation. Men in slaughter houses, truck drivers, hostlers, cattle and horse owners, farmers and stable keepers, may be taken care of by general legislation; but educated men, devoted to scientific research, and physicians, devoted to the relief of suffering humanity, need some special supervision and regulation! Unprejudiced people naturally inquire after the right and the wrong of this matter. Hearing accusations of wantonly cruel deeds actuated by no higher motive than passing curiosity, brought against workers in laboratories and teachers in class-rooms, at first they may be moved to believe that additional special legislation is required. Further thought leads, however, to a further question: If these charges of cruelty are justified, why are not those guilty of it brought up for trial in accordance with the laws already provided against cruelty to animals? Consideration of the fact that the remedies and punishment already provided are not resorted to by those so vehement in their charges against scientific workers leads the unprejudiced inquirer to a further conclusion. Agitation for new laws is not so much intended to prevent specific instances of cruelty to animals as to subject scientific inquiry to hampering restrictions. The moral issue changes to this question: What ought to be the moral attitude of the public to the proposal to put scientific inquiry under restrictive conditions? No one who really asks himself this question, (without mixing it up with the other question of cruelty to animals that is taken care of by already existing laws), can, I imagine, be in doubt as to its answer. Nevertheless, one consideration should be emphasized. *Scientific in-*

quiry has been the chief instrumentality in bringing man from barbarism to civilization, from darkness to light; while it has incurred, at every step, determined opposition from the powers of ignorance, misunderstanding, and jealousy. It is not so long ago, as years are reckoned, that a scientist in a physical or chemical laboratory was popularly regarded as a magician engaged in unlawful pursuits, or as in impious converse with evil spirits, about whom all sorts of detrimental stories were circulated and believed. Those days have gone; generally speaking, the value of free scientific inquiry as an instrumentality of social progress and enlightenment is acknowledged. At the same time, it is still possible, by making irrelevant emotional appeals and obscuring the real issues, to galvanize into life something of the old spirit of misunderstanding, envy, and dread of science. The point at issue in the subjection of animal experimenters to special supervision and legislation is thus deeper than at first sight appears: In principle, it involves the revival of that animosity to discovery and to the application to life of the fruits of discovery which, upon the whole, has been the chief foe of human progress. It behooves every thoughtful individual to be constantly on the alert against every revival of this spirit, in whatever guise it presents itself.

Many "mild" antivivisectionists really object only to the experimental use of animals commonly used as pets, especially dogs and cats. The great majority of animals used in pharmaceutical research are mice and rats, and there does not seem to be too much objection to their use. The survey mentioned earlier indicated that only about one of 260 animals used in research in the ethical pharmaceutical industry in 1968 was a dog; about one in 600 was a cat.

Many Americans have been concerned by charges that significant numbers of research animals, especially dogs and cats, are stolen animals sold to laboratories by unscrupulous dealers. Some witnesses testifying at Congressional hearings have suggested that more than half of all dogs and cats used in research laboratories are stolen. There seems to be a singular lack of evidence for this high incidence, however. Mr. William Mapel, administrative vice president of the American Society for the Prevention of Cruelty to Animals, testifying before a house committee in September, 1965, stated that "over the last several decades . . . the ASPCA has sought to trace and substantiate scores of informal and sometimes anonymous contentions that there is widespread thievery and sale of animals to scientific laboratories. . . . Such investigations have never substantiated or justified official action by the ASPCA in New York, but you may be assured we should be eager to lodge such a complaint and make it stick." For what it is worth, in my quarter of a century in the pharmaceutical research community I have not known personally of a single case in which a stolen animal found its way into our laboratories.

On August 24, 1966, the 89th Congress enacted the Laboratory Animal Welfare Act into law. It had two purposes: 1) to protect owners of dogs and cats from theft of their pets, and 2) to provide humane treatment of certain animals intended for use in research laboratories. Not all research animals are included in the Act. Specifically, it applies only to dogs, cats, nonhuman primates, guinea pigs, hamsters, and rabbits. Mice, rats, pigs, and chickens, among others, are not included, interestingly. The nonhuman primates are members of the highest order of mammals, such as the tiny marmosets, weighing ounces; monkeys, weighing pounds; and the huge gorillas, weighing hundreds of pounds.

Regulations implementing the new Act were issued on February 24, 1967, by the Secretary of Agriculture. The group within the Department of Agriculture to administer these regulations is the Agricultural Research Service of the Animal Health Division. The regulations do *not* apply to animals during actual research or experimentation. The care of animals during these stages is determined by the scientists in the research facility itself. The regulations do establish minimal standards governing housing facilities, including specifications for the sites of cages, pens, or other primary enclosures; feeding; watering; sanitation; ventilation; pest controls; separation by species; veterinary care; and transportation.

A dealer who sells cats and dogs is required to obtain a license from the Secretary of Agriculture by applying to the Veterinarian in Charge in the state in which he operates. Research facilities are not licensed, but they must register with the Secretary by filing proper forms with the Veterinarian in Charge. Dogs and cats sold by dealers must be identified by the use of an official tag or tattoo marking. Complete records for each such animal must be kept for at least one year and longer if requested by the Secretary or his representative. In order to expedite the search for lost or stolen dogs or cats, the law provides for inspection of animals and of records of research facilities and dealers. Dealers are not permitted to sell dogs or cats for at least five business days after acquisition.

Research facilities and governmental agencies may purchase covered animals intended for research only from licensed dealers, persons specifically exempted from the licensing requirement (those who derive less than a substantial part of their income from the breeding and rearing of dogs or cats on their own premises), or from city dog pounds and similar institutions. Dealers who violate the provisions of the Act may have their licenses suspended. If the Secretary of Agriculture finds a research facility to be in violation, he may issue a cease and desist order. If the facility knowingly fails to obey the order, it may be fined $500 for each day of such offense. Orders of the Secretary may, if the dealer or research facility institutes legal action, be reviewed within 60 days in the local federal court.

I have talked with persons who have supposed that animal experimentation can be conducted without causing pain or discomfort to the animals. Unfortunately, this is usually not true. Surgery, of course, is conducted under anesthesia, but only a few experiments involve surgery. When a potential new drug is given to an animal, it may cause pain and discomfort if the animal is not anesthetized. In most cases, anesthesia cannot be used because it would prevent a useful test. Acute toxicity studies involve giving enough compound to kill some of the animals. In chronic studies, the substance is given daily for many months; usually at least one level of dosage produces measurable toxicity, and undoubtedly discomfort often is caused by lower dosage. It would not be possible to detect some targeted activities (for example, analgesia, sedation, tranquilization) if the animals were anesthetized. As a generality, any experiment lasting more than a few hours cannot be done under anesthesia. After all, the animal, at the least, must eat to survive. Finally, even when the response under test can be measured in both normal and anesthetized animals, often it differs qualitatively and quantitatively in the two situations.

Most of the tests in the primary animal screening program seek a "yes" or "no" answer to some definite question. Does the compound lower blood pressure? Does it produce anesthesia? Is it active against an animal infection? Is it active in a test thought to be predictive of some clinical activity? Most laboratories have at least one or two more general primary testing procedures, however. One of these often consists of a number of careful observations of an animal's behavior after he has received the new compound, and usually uses mice or rats. In the Warner-Lambert Research Institute, new substances are given

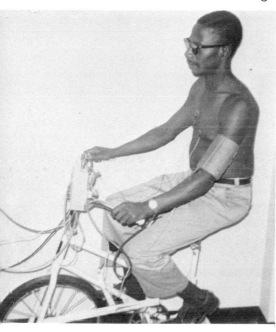

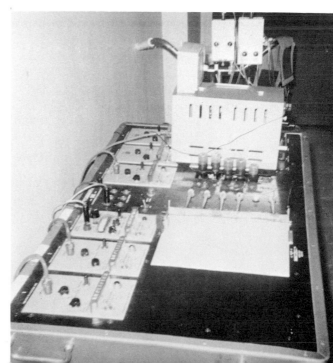

The young man on the
cycle has received an ex-
perimental drug that will
useful, hopefully, in the
treatment of heart disease.
The apparatus in the lower
picture measures heart and
respiratory rate, blood pressure, and electrocardiagram
during exercise. (W-LRI)

by mouth to male rats (two animals for each level of dosage); a trained technician then looks for 42 possible behavior patterns, ranging from ataxia (inability to walk) to death. Is there underactivity or overactivity? If a horse hair is flicked across the cornea of the eye, does the eye blink? If the inside of the ear is tickled, is the head moved away? If the animal appears immobilized, will he right himself if he is placed on his side? Does he assume a bizarre posture? Is there twitching of muscles? Do his eyes protrude? Is his breathing audible? And so on through the long list.

This type of test will at the least detect the presence or absence of biologic activity at the level of dosage tested. At best, it may predict that the compound has activity suggestive of one of the following: tranquilizer, sedative, hypnotic (sleep-producing drug), convulsant, antidepressant, stimulant, strong analgesic (like morphine), muscle relaxant, or vasodilator. If the compound is a potent diuretic (stimulates the flow of urine) the frequency of urination may be increased markedly, although rats, like other animals, often urinate as a result of excitement. Sometimes, if there is bleeding, the new substance may prove to be an anticoagulant (agent that inhibits blood clotting).

One concern of many in research management in the pharmaceutical industry is whether the large amount and duration of toxicity testing of a new drug prior to marketing (and with some drugs, such as contraceptive tablets, for years after marketing) is necessary or justified. If through toxicity testing the chances of encountering unacceptable toxicity in man truly are decreased, it is worth the price in manpower, time and money. But this remains to be proved by experience. Actually the record of the past is not bad in this regard. Paul de Haen has compiled a list of drug entities withdrawn from the market because of unacceptable toxicity for the period 1958 through

1966; it contains only 10 drugs. (Two hundred ninety one entities were marketed during this period.) All these drugs had been marketed prior to 1962, one as early as 1952.

This list really can be shortened, because in three cases the toxicity observed was agranulocytosis (a serious disease in which the white blood cells are decreased), which in man appears due to a hypersensitivity to the drug. Only a few sensitive patients exhibited the reaction, and it is impossible at present to reproduce the condition in animals. In other words, no amount of animal experimentation could have predicted this type of toxicity. In brief, then, about 2.4 percent of the new drug entities marketed during the years 1958-1966 thus far have exhibited toxicity (theoretically detectable in the laboratory) serious enough to cause the drug's removal from the market. Will the record of the next ten years be better? I am inclined to doubt it.

Cats with implanted electrodes are used for site of action studies as well as to evaluate anticonvulsive effect. Responses to electrical stimuli are picked up by antennae, which relay results directly into computers. (II-LAR INC.)

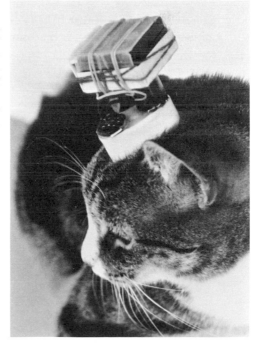

CHAPTER 8

Human Guinea Pigs

Ethics. Principles.
Methodology

A FEW CENTURIES AGO, experimentation on human beings, or even on cadavers, was questioned and often condemned. Apparently, however, this condemnation did not extend to the use of all sorts of mixtures that were administered as potential therapeutic agents. Most of those mixtures that have been recorded in medical history seem ridiculous, or even dangerous, to the modern physician. A few of them have survived, although usually in a purified form—digitalis, quinine, and reserpine, for example. One of the most definitive statements of a code of ethics for human experimentation in more recent times was that made by the famous French physiologist and pioneer of experimental medicine, Claude Bernard (1813-1878).

> So, among the experiments that may be tried on man, those that can only harm are forbidden; those that are innocent are permissible; and those that may do good are obligatory.
> The principle of medical morality consists, then, in never performing on a man an experiment which can be harmful to him in any degree whatsoever, although the result may be of great interest to science—that is, of benefit to save the health of others.

In a sense, the modern physician often does experiment with humans; for example, he may vary the dosage of a drug, or even test a series of drugs, in attempting to find an optimal therapeutic regimen for his patient. So long as he uses accepted drugs in accepted dosages, however, no one thinks of this as true experimentation or as a procedure that requires a special code of ethics.

The civilized world was shocked by the revelations of the Nuremberg trials, held following World War II. Investigations by the Allied Governments uncovered evidence of human experimentation in Nazi Germany so cruel and so casual as to suggest that those scientists who had engaged in it knew no moral limits. This inhuman experimentation on humans took place in a country in which animal experimentation was forbidden. Seven of the Nazi defendants, including four physicians, were hanged in 1948 and nine others received prison sentences. In rendering its judgment, the military tribunal wrote a tenpoint code for permissible experimentation on humans. In doing so, it was assumed that human experimentation is justified when it is designed to obtain results for the good of society that could not be obtained in any other way. In 1964, at a meeting of the World Medical Association in Helsinki, Finland, a code of ethics, enlarging on the earlier one resulting from the Nuremberg trials, was adopted. This Declaration of Helsinki, as it is termed, was endorsed by the House of Delegates of the American Medical Association in 1966. The important recommendations of the Declaration of Helsinki are:

I. BASIC PRINCIPLES

1. Clinical research must conform to the moral and scientific principles that justify medical research and should be based on laboratory and animal experiments or other scientifically established facts.

2. Clinical research should be conducted only by scientifically qualified persons and under the supervision of a qualified medical man.

3. Clinical research cannot legitimately be carried out unless the importance of the objective is in proportion to the inherent risk to the subject.

4. Every clinical research project should be preceded by careful assessment of inherent risks in comparison to forseeable benefits to the subject or to others.

5. Special caution should be exercised by the doctor in performing clinical research in which the personality of the subject is liable to be altered by drugs or experimental procedure.

II. CLINICAL RESEARCH COMBINED WITH PROFESSIONAL CARE

1. In the treatment of the sick person, the doctor must be free to use a new therapeutic measure, if in his judgment it offers hope of saving life, reestablishing health, or alleviating suffering.

If at all possible, consistent with patient psychology, the doctor should obtain the patient's freely given consent after the patient has been given a full explanation. In case of legal incapacity, consent should also be procured from the legal guardian; in case of physical incapacity the permission of the legal guardian replaces that of the patient.

2. The doctor can combine clinical research with professional care, the objective being the acquisition of new medical knowledge, only to the extent that clinical research is justified by its therapeutic value for the patient.

III. NONTHERAPEUTIC CLINICAL RESEARCH

1. In the purely scientific application of clinical research carried out on the human being, it is the duty of

the doctor to remain the protector of the life and health of that person on whom clinical research is being carried out.

2. The nature, the purpose, and the risk of clinical research must be explained to the subject by the doctor.

3a. Clinical research on a human being cannot be undertaken without his free consent after he has been informed; if he is legally incompetent, the consent of the legal guardian should be procured.

3b. The subject of clinical research should be in such a mental, physical, and legal state as to be able to exercise fully his power of choice.

3c. Consent should, as a rule, be obtained in writing. However, the responsibility for clinical research always remains with the research worker; it never falls on the subject even after consent is obtained.

4a. The investigator must respect the right of each individual to safeguard his personal integrity, especially if the subject is in a dependent relationship to the investigator.

4b. At any time during the course of clinical research, the subject or his guardian should be free to withdraw permission for research to be continued.

The investigator or the investigating team should discontinue the research if in his or their judgment, it may, if continued, be harmful to the individual.

The Declaration of Helsinki is not, of course, a legal document; it is, quite simply, a guide for physicians and others engaged in research in which humans are the experimental subjects. The principle that the patient or subject should as a rule consent to the experiment, however, is written into the Kefauver-Harris Amendments of 1962. This act provides that regulations to be issued impose the condition that investigators "obtain the consent of such human beings or their representatives, except where they deem it is not feasible or, in their professional judgment, contrary to the best interests of such human beings." Regulations implementing this, issued in final form on June 20, 1967, in part state:

> . . . the consent of such humans (or the consent of their representatives) to whom investigational drugs are administered primarily for the accumulation of scientific knowledge, for such purposes as studying drug behavior, body processes, or the course of a disease, must be obtained in all cases and in all but exceptional cases, the consent of patients under treatment with investigational drugs or the consent of their representatives must be obtained.

The three phases of clinical trials defined in the FDA regulations were discussed in Chapter 2. In Phase 1, the experimental drug is given to well or sick humans, not chiefly as a therapeutic agent but for the purpose of obtaining more information about its pharmacologic action in man. All of the subjects used in Phase 1 investigations must consent to their participation in the experiment, and this consent *must* be in writing.

In Phase 2 studies, in which the drug is used as a therapeutic agent in a limited number of patients, consent is required, but some exceptions to this requirement are permitted.

> For example, where the patient is in a coma or is otherwise incapable of giving informed consent, his representatives cannot be reached, and it is imperative to administer the drug without delay.

Another exception might be a situation in which the physician, ordinarily with the concurrence of the family—perhaps also of the patient's spiritual advisor—believes it is contrary to the best interest of his patient to disclose the nature of his illness to him. The patient might, for instance, have a fatal illness and might be of such a temperament that disclosure of this fact to him would cause a mental breakdown. If it were necessary to describe the illness in the course of obtaining "informed consent" from such patient, the physician could be justified in giving the experimental drug without the patient's consent. Of course, in the example cited, the family would know the physician's plans and would concur. If, however, no representative of the patient were available, the physician would use his own best judgment in deciding whether to give the drug without consent. Whenever consent is required in Phase 2 studies, it must be in writing.

In Phase 3 investigations, in which the experimental agent is tested in large numbers of patients,

> it is the responsibility of the investigator, taking into consideration the physical and mental state of the patient, to decide when it is necessary or preferable to obtain consent in other than written form. When written consent is not obtained, the investigator must obtain oral consent and record that fact in the medical record of the person receiving the drug.

In exceptional cases, such as those cited for Phase 2 investigations, the drug may be given without consent.

In obtaining consent, the investigator is expected to explain as carefully as possible the reasons for the administration of the experimental drug, the nature of the drug, the expected duration of the experiment, the method of administration, the hazards involved, the existence of alternative forms of therapy, and the possible benefits to the patient that might result from the therapeutic procedure. Admittedly, with many, or even most, patients, it is difficult for the physician to explain all of these things in nonmedical terms so that the patient truly understands them. Moreover, if the drug is new, the physician himself cannot really do more than predict such things as hazards and benefits. All he can do, then, is to insure that the patient's consent is "informed" within the limitations of the patient's ability to understand and his own ability to communicate.

The possible legal liabilities assumed by the physician who administers experimental drugs to patients are not really known. In the past, the courts have used the word "experimentation," but always in the sense of malpractice. That is, they have ruled that the physician has deviated in a significant way from the practice of his colleagues in the same or a similar locality. According to Irving Ladmer, writing in 1960, "the fact is that, to date, there has been no recorded case in which a court has been confronted with clinical evaluation or investigation in the modern sense."

If the investigation involves well persons rather than patients, the potential liability is even more difficult to predict. As a generality, persons who, with full knowledge of the risks involved, voluntarily expose themselves to these risks cannot recover damages for injuries received. In an actual case, presumably the key elements the court would consider would be "knowledge of the risks" and "voluntary choice." The only logical reason for giving experimental drugs to well people is potential social benefit. If litigation should arise, the court must balance this possible social benefit against the risk to the subject.

An investigator, working under the aegis of a sponsor who has filed a proper IND with the FDA might, of course, violate the law. He might, as an example, fail to obtain the consent of subjects in a Phase 1 investigation; or he might submit false information to the sponsor. When either or both of these deficiencies becomes known to the FDA, he will receive written notice from its Director of the Bureau of Medicine, who will offer him the opportunity "to explain the matter in an

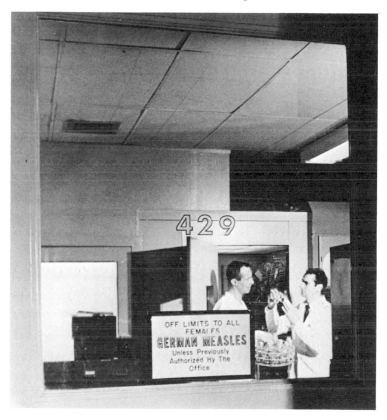

Because German measles infection is hazardous to unborn babies, particularly when the mother is in the first three months of pregnancy, some units of the MS&D Laboratories were made off limits to women. (MS&D)

informal conference and/or in writing." If his explanation is not acceptable, the Commissioner of the FDA will provide the investigator the opportunity for an informal hearing, and if the Commissioner determines that the investigator has repeatedly

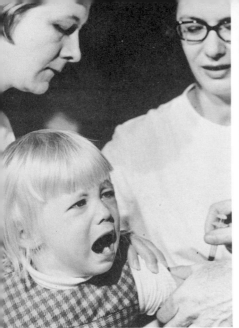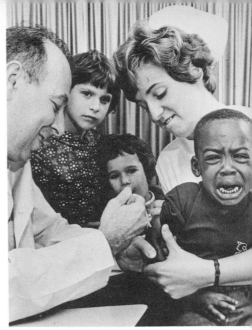

A three-year-old Danbury girl receives her mumps vaccination at a clinic sponsored by the Danbury Hospital and the Yale University School of Medicine, before its licensing early in 1968. The administration at the right took place at the John F. Kennedy Hospital in Philadelphia. During the various studies, more than 6,500 children received vaccinations. (MS&D)

or deliberately failed to comply with the regulations or has submitted false data to the sponsor, and has failed to furnish adequate assurance that his future conduct will be satisfactory, he will then notify the investigator and the sponsor that the investigator is not entitled to receive investigational-use drugs. The data provided to a sponsor by an investigator who has been thus "blacklisted" by the FDA cannot be used to justify continuation of an investigation or in support of an NDA. In extreme cases, this may result in termination of the study of an experimental drug or in the disapproval of an NDA. The validity of these FDA regulations has not been determined by the courts. The investigator may be reinstated as eligible to receive and use investigational-use drugs where the Commissioner finds that he has presented adequate assurance that he will test them in compliance with the regulations and will submit accurate reports to the sponsor.

Each marketed package of a prescription drug contains a printed package insert. This document contains all of the information required for a physician to use the drug intelligently. It is classified as a part of the labeling of the drug by the FDA, and has been approved by that Agency prior to marketing the drug.

If a practicing physician, in the treatment of his patient, deviates from the directions in the package insert, has he been guilty of violating the law? This question arises because the definition of a new drug in the Kefauver-Harris Drug Amendments includes "well known drugs and combinations of drugs bearing label directions for higher dosage or more frequent dosage or for longer duration of use than have become recognized as safe and effective." This wording has been interpreted by the FDA to mean that a marketed drug becomes a "new drug" (at least where clinical experimentation is involved) if the dosage used or the disease treated has not been approved by that Agency.

To restate the problem: Is it illegal for a physician to use a "new drug" as defined in the preceding sentence in the treatment of his patient (as differentiated from the conduct of a clinical investigation) if it is not covered by an approved NDA? Ordinarily this would be done within a single state and, in my opinion (and in the opinions of lawyers with whom I have consulted), there would be no actual violation of the new drug provisions. Suppose, however, he transported the drug across a state line (perhaps from his office in one state to a hospital in an adjoining state). What then?

The FDA has indicated that it has no intention of testing

this in the courts. There has remained the question of how a court would rule on the importance of the package insert in a malpractice suit, although this has been answered recently by the Supreme Judicial Court of Massachusetts. It ruled that the package insert "was no more than a recommendation" and that since (in the case under consideration) there was a difference of opinion among the anesthesiologists over proper dosage, the package insert could not be considered binding.

The great advance in the methodology of testing drugs in humans in recent years has been the widespread use of the controlled experiment. In this type of experiment, the new agent is tested against a placebo (inert material), an established drug, or both, under circumstances in which neither the investigator nor the patient knows which dosage form has been used. Moreover, the experiment has been designed with the assistance of a statistician, and set up in such a way that the results obtained can be analyzed mathematically and the odds that the results obtained are due to chance can be calculated. Also, the experiment has been designed to answer definite questions.

Not too long ago, new drugs usually were sent to investigators who were experts in the disease for which the drug was designed as a therapeutic agent. These investigators gave the drug to a number of their patients and formed impressions of its probable value and potential toxicity. Their reports to the sponsor of the new drug often were only summaries of the experiments together with their conclusions. This type of "open" experiment still is used often in Phase 3 investigations, but only after definitive answers have been obtained by controlled investigations. Moreover, the individual record for each patient studied, even in open studies, is required to be filed in an NDA.

Many diseases fluctuate widely from day to day in their

severity or symptomatology. Open experimentation thus can be misleading: the patient's condition might have changed in spite of—rather than because of—the administration of the new drug. Moreover, many patients are "placebo reactors"; that is, they are suggestible and react favorably when they take a placebo but are under the impression they have been given an active drug. Further, the physician himself is not immune to suggestion, and his judgment of the patient's possible change of clinical state may be biased, albeit unconsciously. .

I remember well my introduction to the power of a placebo. Some years ago, when I was a pharmacist in my home town in Florida, a lady whom I had known most of my life called me on the telephone one day:

"Earle, I am worried about that prescription you filled and sent to me."

"What bothers you, Mrs. S———?"

"Well, as you know, my husband has a broken leg and he has been in great pain. I gave him one of those white capsules you sent. In fifteen minutes the pain was gone and he turned over and went to sleep. I am afraid to give him anything that strong!"

"Mrs. S———, Dr. T——— is a very competent doctor and your husband has been his patient for a long time. He wouldn't prescribe anything harmful and, since I filled the prescription, I can assure you that the medicine in those capsules is not harmful. Just be glad that your husband responded so well."

Now, I could give Mrs. S——— that assurance because I knew that each white capsule contained only 5 grains of common baking soda! Obviously this physician knew his patient.

The type of controlled experiment described above often is referred to as a "double blind" experiment, when a new agent is compared to a placebo. If another drug is included also, the experiment is a "triple blind" one. Of course, even more substances can be included, but limitations of time and the number of patients available usually preclude this. In carrying out controlled experiments, it is important that all of the substances tested (drug or drugs and placebo) be incorporated into identical dosage forms. Usually this is not difficult. Sometimes, however, if the experimental compound has unique physical properties (perhaps it is a liquid with a characteristic odor), this becomes a difficult feat that really tests the skill of the pharmacist who devises the dosage forms.

The objective of controlled studies of new drugs in humans is to gain useful information (at the dosage tested) about efficacy, side effects, toxicity, or all three. *Side effects* are undesirable effects that result from an exaggeration of the biologic properties of a drug. For example, when atropine is given for the purpose of relieving intestinal cramping, an effective dose usually causes, as a side effect, dryness of the mouth. If the dose is increased, the patient may experience other side effects, such as blurring of vision or difficulty in starting a flow of urine. All this is explained by the fact that atropine acts on certain nerves in the body. These nerves go to various tissues and, depending on dosage, atropine can affect any or all of them.

A new drug that causes actual tissue damage is *toxic*, at least in the dosage that caused the damage, which does not necessarily rule out its use as a drug in proper dosage. Also, if the drug is to be used in the therapy of a fatal illness such as cancer, the physician may be willing to accept a great deal of toxicity if the drug benefits his patient. Sometimes the toxicity is related to sensitivity of the patient to the drug. For example, ordinarily penicillin is nontoxic, but occasionally sensitive patients can experience severe reactions if they receive injections of it. Ordinarily, experimental drugs that cause damage to tissues such as the liver, kidney, gastrointestinal tract, brain, or heart are unacceptable unless the toxic dose is far removed from the effective therapeutic dose. Recently we have become aware of the possibility that drugs may affect adversely the development of an unborn child without exhibiting any toxicity in the mother. Thus, experimental drugs are not given to women capable of bearing children (except occasionally to long-term female prisoners) until careful laboratory tests on animals have been completed. These tests were described in Chapter 2.

Several problems should be faced before a controlled experiment is started. What dosage is to be used? One must remember that the results obtained are "true" for that dosage only; different results may be obtained if the experiment is repeated at a different dosage. What questions do we wish to answer? They might be, for example: What percentage of patients with a specified involvement of chronic osteoarthritis obtain some measurable degree of relief from the use of the new drug? How does this compare with the percentage who obtain the same degree of relief by taking a certain dosage of aspirin? Do patients taking the new drug experience more or fewer side effects than those taking aspirin? Does either aspirin or the new drug give more positive responses than the placebo?

In addition, the acceptable "p value" (probability value) for each question must be decided. A p value of 0.05, which means the calculated probability that the result obtained is due to chance is 5 in 100 (or 1 in 20), often is regarded as indicating statistical significance. On the other hand, for some types of drug it might be desirable that the p value be 0.01 (odds are 1 to 100 that the result is due to chance) or less. In this case, usually many more patients must be studied than for the first group, in order to obtain enough information to justify this conclusion. In still other cases, lower p values (say 0.1 or 0.2) might be regarded as indicating *possible* activity so that further study is justified.

An actual example may be helpful in illustrating some of these points. In this experiment, an experimental drug designed to induce sleep in patients with insomnia was compared with a placebo in a double blind study. Approximately 1,000 patients were included, of whom half received the experimental drug and half received placebo. A single dose of the drug was given at bedtime; the questions asked involved the patients' subjective evaluations of onset, quality, and duration of sleep, and whether they felt rested and wide awake on arousal. The answers obtained from the study were as follows:

1. The incidence of sleep occurring in less than 30 minutes for patients receiving the drug was 35 percent, and for those receiving the placebo, 27 percent. The calculated p value was 0.06. In other words the odds were 6 in 100 that this difference might have been due to chance and not to an actual difference between the two agents.

2. The incidence of good to excellent sleep in those subjects receiving the drug was 70 percent; for those receiving the placebo 48 percent. This difference was highly significant, since the calculated p value was 0.001—that is, only 1 chance in 1,000 that the difference was due to chance.

3. The percentage of patients reporting less than 6 hours of sleep was 27 percent of those taking the drug and 45 percent of those taking the placebo. The difference again was highly significant since the calculated p value was 0.002—that is, odds of 2 in 1,000 that the difference was due to chance.

4. Seventy-two percent of those taking the drug felt rested and wide awake on arousal, 60 percent of the placebo group. The difference was significant at the 0.02 level (the odds were 2 in 100 that the difference was due to chance).

It is worth making special note of the apparent results obtained with the placebo. If only placebo, and no drug, had been given, an unsuspecting investigator of an earlier generation might have concluded that the placebo was a useful drug. It is not always useful or even desirable to use placebos and double or triple blind tests. In Phase 1 studies, the investigator usually works only with the new agent. He is concerned with its pharmacologic activity in man and its possible effects on target organs such as the liver, kidney, and heart. Often studies of absorption and excretion of the drug or its end products are made. Studies of this type do not require that some second substance be used as a control.

In other cases, the type of drug makes it impossible, or at least undesirable, to give some of the patients a placebo. This is true, for example, in the evaluation of a new drug designed to prevent conception. Two active contraceptive drugs could be compared double-blind fashion with each other, of course, but if both truly were effective, little if any difference would be found. If large numbers of patients were used, this type of study might give useful information about differences in side effects or toxicity. The treatment of a potentially fatal acute infection is another situation in which it is not practical to use the double blind technic, at least if it involves the administration of a placebo. In fact, the investigator must be prepared to stop the use of the experimental drug and to institute therapy with a standard drug at a moment's notice if it becomes evident that the new agent is not effective.

In Phase 3 investigations, after efficacy and toxicity have been evaluated carefully in controlled experiments, the drug may be given to large numbers of patients in open studies. The objective is to gain some insight into its behavior as a therapeutic agent when it is used, as it will be later, in actual clinical practice.

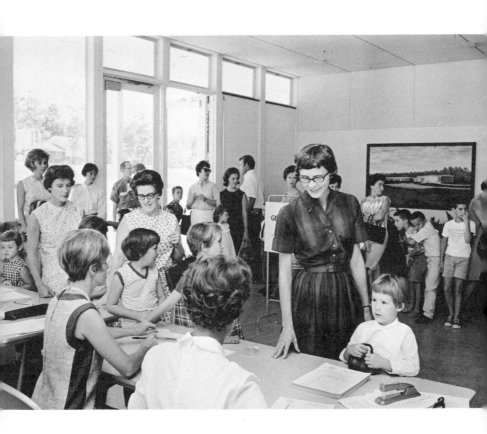

This German measles field trial, in Danbury, Connecticut, helped insure the effectiveness of rubella vaccine before it was licensed by HEW in June, 1969. (MS&D)

CHAPTER 9

Patents and Drugs

Patent History, Law, Value.
Government Policy. For Reform.
Trademarks. Copyrights

Lɛᴛᴛᴇʀs ᴘᴀᴛᴇɴᴛ, a compound noun that has been used for centuries, is derived from the Latin words, *litterae patentes*, meaning "open letters," or more broadly, "written documents open to scrutiny by the public." *Webster's Third New International Dictionary, Unabridged,* defines *letter patent* as follows:

> Written communication usually signed and sealed from a government or sovereign of a nation conferring upon a designated person a grant (as a right, title, status, property, authority, privilege, monopoly, franchise, immunity, or exemption) that could not otherwise be enjoyed in a form readily open for inspection by all seeking confirmation of the grant conferred.

The United States Patent Office defines a patent as a "grant issued by the United States Government giving an inventor the right to exclude all others from making, using, or selling his invention within the United States, its territories and possessions" for a period of seventeen years. That is, of course, the grant of a monoply, although in something of a negative sense. The holder of a patent really is not given an absolute right to do anything, but he is granted the right to prevent others from doing something—from practicing his invention during the life of the patent.

Even more important to society, perhaps, is that the patent

gives a complete disclosure of the invention to the public. Other inventors, engineers, and scientists thus can make use of this information in planning investigations that may result in valuable new discoveries. If it were not for the protection given by the patent, the inventor usually would be forced to exploit his invention secretly in order to gain maximal benefit for himself. It is known that letters patent, or patents, were granted in Venice as early as 1474. At various times thereafter, they were granted by governments or sovereigns, but a regular legal system providing for the grant of patents in the modern sense did not exist before 1623. England then passed a law designed to abolish commercial monopolies, but provided a specific exemption, however, for inventions:

> Provided, nevertheless, and be it declared and enacted: That any declaration before mentioned shall not extend to any letters patent and grants of privilege, for the term of one and twenty years or under, heretofore made of the sole working or making of any manner of new manufacture, within this realm, to the first and true inventor or inventors of such manufacture, which others, at the time of the making of such letters patent and grants did not use, so they be not contrary to the law, nor mischievous to the state. . . .

Some patents were granted by the American colonies. Usually exclusive rights were given only when it was obvious that doing so would be profitable to the colony. The effective period of exclusivity was brief, and a special act of the legislature was required for each patent. In general, the legislature was more concerned about benefit to the public than to the inventor. When the United States constitution was adopted, it contained a provision for the establishment of a patent system.

> The Congress shall have the Power . . . To promote the

Progress of Science and useful Arts, by securing for limited Times to Authors and Inventors the exclusive Right to their respective Writings and Discoveries. . . .

Congress passed the first Patent Act in 1790, which stipulated that patents would be granted for "any useful art, manufacture, engine, machine, or device, or any improvement thereon not before known or used." The first patent issued under the new law was granted to Samuel Hopkins of Philadelphia for an improvement in "the making of Pot ash and Pearl ash by a new Apparatus and Process."

The responsibility for granting patents was given to a Board consisting of the Secretary of State, the Secretary of War, and the Attorney General; responsibility for administering the law was given to the Department of State. Patents were to be issued for variable periods of time, not to exceed 14 years. Samuel Hopkins' patent was signed by George Washington, President of the United States, Edmund Randolph, Attorney General, and Thomas Jefferson, Secretary of State. The original signed document is preserved in the collections of the Chicago Historical Society.

In 1793, the Patent Act was changed drastically. The new act deleted the requirement that an invention be "sufficiently useful and important," and as a result, applications no longer were examined for novelty and usefulness. Patents simply were granted to those who applied for them, submitted proper drawings, and paid the necessary fee. This unfortunate system remained in effect until July 4, 1836, when a new Patent Act was passed, which reestablished the "examination" system in effect before 1793. Patents were to be issued only if novelty and usefulness had been established, and once again the "prior art"—that which had been used or discovered before—must be searched in order to establish that the claimed invention indeed was new. Our present patent laws are based on the principles set forth in this law. Patents issued prior to the Act of 1836 were not numbered. The first numbered patent (1) was issued on July 13, 1836, to John Ruggles, Senator from Maine, for an implement "designed to give a multiplied tractive power to the locomotive and to prevent the evil of the sliding of the wheels."

At first, the Patent Office was established as a bureau within the Department of State. On March 3, 1849, it was transferred to the newly created Department of the Interior, and finally, on April 1, 1925, to its present organizational niche in the Department of Commerce.

Under the United States patent system the basic requirements are that the claimed invention shall be new and useful and that it shall be the discovery of a first and original inventor. An issued patent is property owned by the inventor. He may grant licenses to others to practice the invention or a specified portion of it; he is not obligated, of course, to grant such licenses. He may assign the patent to other individuals or to a legal establishment, such as a business enterprise or a nonprofit corporation. Patents also may be dedicated to the government or to the public. The inventor has the right to sell the patent if he wishes; in such case, the purchaser has the full rights previously possessed by the inventor.

When a patent application reaches the Patent Office, it is referred to a patent examiner. His first task is to decide whether or not the claimed invention really is novel—that is, that it has not been known previously to those "versed in the art." To determine this, he searches the patent and scientific literature. If he finds a previous disclosure closely related to the claims in the patent application, he must make a judgment: is the previous disclosure sufficient to make the presently claimed invention something that would be obvious to anyone skilled in the art? If the invention, for example, is a new chemical compound that has analgesic activity, would a trained medicinal chemist know that if he made the new compound it would have this type of activity? Obviously a judgment must be made. It is fairly certain in the case of the example cited, however, that a true invention has been made. Predictions of the biologic activities of new chemical substances more often than not prove wrong. Hence, the finding of the claimed biologic activity for the new compound represents a discovery of something new (the compound) and useful (the biologic activity). Judge Learned Hand has made this comment about the problem of deciding whether a claimed discovery represents patentable inventiveness:

> An invention is a new display of ingenuity beyond the compass of the routineer, and in the end that is all that can be said about it. Courts cannot avoid the duty of divining as best they can what the day to day capacity of the ordinary artisan will produce. This they attempt by looking at the history of the art, the occasion for the invention, its success, its independent repetition at about the same time, and the state of the underlying art, which was a condition upon its appearance at all. Yet, when all is said, there will remain cases when we can only fall back upon such good sense as we may have, and in these we cannot help exposing the inventor to the hazard inherent in hypostatizing such modifications in the existing arts as are within the limited imagination of the journeyman. There comes a point when the question must be resolved by a subjective opinion as to what seems an easy step and what does not. We must try to correct our standard by such objective references as we can, but in the end the judgment will appear, and no doubt be, to a large extent personal, and in that sense arbitrary.

The second requirement for patentability of an invention

is that it be useful. The Patent Office has published guidelines that it believes will be helpful in deciding whether a new drug meets this requirement.

Utility must be definite and in currently available form; not merely for further investigation or research. Thus generalized and vague assertions such as "therapeutic agents," "for pharmacological purposes," "biological activity," "intermediates," and for making further unspecified preparations are regarded as too nebulous and insufficient.

If the specified or implied utility involves humans, clinical evidence is necessary; however, there is authority that animal tests are acceptable if the tests are of a kind that the results are known to be closely correlated with human utility. In accordance with the present case law, if there is no assertion of human utility, operativeness for use on standard test animals is adequate for patent purposes. Further, if the evidence shows that the drug is not safe in the dosage or mode of use for which it is effective, the disclosure will not satisfy the utility requirement. . . . Absolute safety is not necessarily required.

The standards of disclosure . . . in respect to the statutory language of "written description of . . . using" the invention "as to enable any person skilled in the art to which it pertains . . . to use the same" are to be strictly construed in view of the special public interest involved. Thus the extension of specific utilities to classes of compounds must be adequately supported by sufficient and typical exemplification and by a representation that the class as a whole possesses the asserted utility.

In the case of mixtures formulated including a drug as an ingredient or mixtures which are drugs or methods of treating a specific condition with a drug, whether old or new, a specific example of how to use must be set forth, which will include the organism treated and the mode and parameters of administration.

The third requirement is that a patent be granted only to the first inventor. Now it sometimes happens that two or more persons will file patent applications containing claims that describe essentially the same invention. When this occurs, the Patent Office must try to determine who is, in fact, the first inventor. The patent examiner proceeds by rewriting the similar claims so that they are identical. He then forwards his files to the examiner of interferences, and the Commissioner of Patents notifies the parties involved that an interference exists. The parties then submit testimony in writing to the Patent Office. Usually the junior party (the senior party is the first party that filed an application) submits testimony first. If it does not establish that the junior party made the invention prior to the filing date of the senior party, the interference is terminated, as the application of the junior party is also. If it turns out that the junior party did, in fact, make the invention prior to the filing date of the senior party, testimony from the senior party also is sent to the Patent Office. The case then is argued orally before the Board of Interference Examiners. This Board decides which person is the original inventor and therefore entitled to the patent. This decision can be appealed, however, to the Court of Customs and Patent Appeals, or either applicant may elect to appeal to another federal court, such as the District Court of the District of Columbia.

An interference also can be created by an inventor who believes that an issued patent contains a claim or claims that he believes cover an invention made independently by himself. To do this, he files a new application containing a claim or claims identical with the one or more of those of the issued patent. This must be done within one year from the date of the issuance of the patent. The interference procedure already described then is set up by the Patent Office.

The determination of the date of the original invention again involves difficult decisions of judgment. Usually the inventor will have made a written "concept of invention" as his first step in pursuing the invention. The next important date is that on which he began to reduce this concept to practice. A chemist, for example, may write down a chemical structure, or a series of chemically related structures. In a properly managed research laboratory, this concept will be dated and witnessed by another chemist capable of understanding the proposed chemistry. At a later date, the chemist searches the literature, orders necessary chemical intermediates, and prepares to attempt the preparation of the new compounds; finally, he makes them and submits them for biologic testing. If one of them is sufficiently potent and nontoxic, it will be tested in humans. Presumably, all of these events will have been recorded, dated, and witnessed by scientists capable of understanding the scientific procedures involved.

Now, it may happen that one person has the earliest date of conception, whereas the second party has the earliest date of actual reduction to practice. Usually the Patent Office has ruled that the person who first reduced the invention to practice is the true inventor, but this has not always been so.

A patent application has certain formal parts: the petition, the specification and claims, the oath, and the official filing fee. The specification is a discussion of the invention, and usually includes examples "in such full, clear, concise, and exact terms as to enable any person skilled in the art . . . to make, construct, compound, and use the same." The statute requires that the inventor "shall particularly point out and distinctly claim the particular improvement or combination which is claimed as his invention or discovery." Often the inventor states the objects of the invention in the specification. After the nature of the invention is discussed in the specification, definite numbered claims, defining as exactly as possible the scope of the invention, are appended. Material given in the specification but not included in the claims belongs to the public and not to the inventor. As examples of the way in which claims may be worded, two of the claims in the patent covering epinephrine (adrenaline), the first hormone to be purified and marketed, are cited:

1. A substance possessing the herein-described physiological characteristics and reactions of the suprarenal glands in a stable and concentrated form, and practically free from inert and associated gland-tissue.

6. A crystalline substance possessing the herein-described physiological characteristics and reactions of the suprarenal glands; said substances having the property of crystallizing in a variety of forms.

Several types of claim may be obtained in patents involving drugs. The most valuable is a product claim, in which the new drug, or a new chemical series of compounds, is claimed as the invention. But if the drug itself is old and not patentable, a new method of manufacture may be the only invention specified in the claims. Of course a competitor could avoid a "method" claim by devising an alternative procedure for making the drug, and method claims may be included in patents that have new product claims.

Sometimes mixtures of drugs exhibit unexpected clinical utility, in which event the combination may be patentable, whether the drugs themselves are old or new. A use, as contrasted with a product or a machine, is not patentable; however, sometimes a method can be patented if it involves the use of a product, even though the product itself may be old. For example, it might be possible to obtain allowance of a claim involving the use of a specified mixture of antibiotics when the mixture is injected intravenously or intramuscularly in the treatment of a specific disease. This type of claim would only be granted, of course, if it represented a true invention. A "use" claim of this type has the disadvantage that the individual who might violate it would be the physician or nurse who administered the drug. Such a claim would probably prevent, on the other hand, a competitor from describing the patented method in its literature, even if the drugs themselves were old. If it did so, it could be sued by the owner of the patent on the grounds of "contributory infringement." In some cases, new dosage forms can be patented, and new machines used in producing drugs, or in packaging them, often can be patented also.

If a patent application is rejected by the examiner, the applicant has the right of appeal to the Board of Appeals. If this Board sustains the examiner, the applicant can then appeal to the Court of Customs and Patent Appeals in Washington, or he may file an original bill in equity (similar to an appeal) before the District Court of the District of Columbia. The advantage of the latter procedure is that new evidence and witnesses may be presented to the court, whereas in procedures before the Court of Customs and Patent Appeals, no evidence except that considered by the Board of Appeals can be introduced. Discoveries that are published in the scientific literature cannot be patented unless an application is filed within one year of publication. If the object of the patent application has been offered for sale or prior public use more than one year before the application, a patent cannot be granted.

I believe it is true that most students of American history agree that much of the credit for the tremendous rate of progress in the industrial arts in this country since 1790 must be given to the patent system. Inventors have been encouraged by it to risk their time and money in making useful and profitable inventions. Today big business furnishes much of the capital required to exploit patented inventions. It may be surprising to learn, however, that about 25 percent of all patents issued today go to individuals. About half the patents granted to private industry go to small companies, a sizeable figure, since private industry receives about 70 percent of the patents issued. Some important discoveries described in patents issued to individual inventors are the Polaroid camera, the vacuum tube, air conditioning, xerography, power steering, DDT, the helicopter, metallic titanium, the self-winding wristwatch, the zipper, FM radio, the gyrocompass, automatic transmissions, and the antibiotics streptomycin and chloramphenicol.

The story of penicillin, briefly told in Chapter 3, is a good example of what may happen when an inventor outside of industry makes a valuable discovery but neglects to patent it. Sir Alexander Fleming apparently was not aware of the value of a patent as an incentive to the development of a marketed product. Moreover, he thought it would be unseemly for a university scientist to patent a discovery that he wished to dedicate to the public. Thus his discovery was made in 1929, but penicillin did not become available even to the armed forces until 1943. Its development by government and industry in the United States might well have been slower if it had not become an urgent war-time project. In later years, Sir Alexander recognized that he had made a mistake in not patenting his discovery. In an article, "Penicillin in Perspective," prepared in 1958, he wrote:

> I have had a great extension of my experiences as the result of penicillin. There is only one serious regret that I have about the whole affair. That is that I did not, on behalf of my colleagues and the laboratory, patent the processes by which penicillin was extracted. This, look-

ing back on it, was a cardinal error, but at that time patenting of medicinal substances by medically qualified people was heavily frowned upon both in Great Britain and the United States.

Back in 1900, after a Japanese commissioner had visited Washington in order to study our patent system, he stated: "We have looked about us to see what nations are the greatest, so that we can be like them. . . . We said, 'What is it that makes the United States such a great nation?' and we investigated and found that it was patents, and we will have patents."

The rate of discovery and marketing of drugs in countries having good patent systems, and in the United States in particular, is far higher than in Italy, countries behind the Iron Curtain, and other countries with weak or nonexistent patent protection for drugs. The five most advanced industrial countries of the world—the United States, Germany, Japan, England, and France—have had patent systems for years. The value of the patent system generally is recognized throughout the free world; for example, the European Common Market presently is engaged in working out a common system of product patents for pharmaceuticals.

The ethical pharmaceutical industry in the United States spent about $400 million in research and development during 1966; the average number of new drug entities marketed annually during the years 1962-1967 was 20. What was the cost per new entity? The answer to this question depends on how we make the calculation. It might be assumed that the discovery and marketing of a new entity is the major aim of ethical drug research; if so, a rough estimate of cost could be made by dividing $400 million by 20, and on this basis, the cost of a new entity would be $20 million. On the other hand, the total number of ethical drugs (including 15 duplicate single products) marketed in 1966 was 80; if the $400 million is divided by 80, the cost per drug comes out to be $5 million.

A fairer way of estimating the cost of a new drug entity, perhaps, is to accumulate the costs involved in its discovery, study in the laboratory, and clinical evaluation, which involves the costs of making the series of synthetic chemicals of which one was chosen for development, the costs of the necessary physical and analytical procedures, and of chemical development; the costs of pharmacologic, physiologic, microbiologic, biochemical, toxicologic, and pathologic studies; the costs of pharmaceutical investigations (making dosage forms, doing stability studies, devising quality control and manufacturing procedures); the costs of clinical investigations; the costs of supporting services (such as statistics, library, graphic arts and technical information services, project planning, medical writing, new personnel, and so on). I am not aware that this type of calculation has been made with any degree of accuracy. If it were done, I am sure that the resulting figure would be several million dollars. The Pharmaceutical Manufacturers Association (who did not use this detailed method of calculation, however) has estimated that an important new drug probably costs about $7 million.

In addition to this cost, the pharmaceutical manufacturer must spend more millions of dollars in distributing the new drug and in the various activities (promotion, advertising, detailing, sampling) that are necessary in order that the practicing physicians in this country will know about the availability of the new drug, its therapeutic indications, the proper dosage and methods of using it, and the potential side effects or toxicity. It seems highly unlikely, at least to me, that a manufacturer would very often be willing to invest this vast amount of money in a new drug if he had no patent protection. Otherwise, within a short period of time, a competitor could market the same drug at a fraction of the cost. In other words, the competitive organization could make a substantial profit even if it sold the new drug at a much lower price than that of the innovator company. This might very well mean that the innovator—who should be rewarded for giving the new drug to the world—in fact will lose money. If this occurred, the incentive to discover more useful drugs might well have been lost.

There are sincere people who argue that patents covering drugs should not be granted. One argument presented is that the cost of developing the new drug by a second company should not differ greatly from the cost of initial development. This conclusion is made because the data submitted by the innovator company in support of its NDA are not available from the FDA for other companies. Obviously, then, similar information must be filed by a second company who submits an NDA. The fallacy to this argument is obvious when one realizes that most of the information in the first NDA will soon appear in the scientific literature. Scientists in the industry and clinical investigators outside insist on the right to publish their scientific investigations; otherwise, they have no way of building a scientific reputation. Most thoughtful people in pharmaceutical management recognize that, on balance, publication of scientific information from the research laboratories is desirable. It enriches the store of scientific information, and it often enables other scientists to make valuable new discoveries. The information published by rival organizations becomes available to all interested scientists.

Now, a second company can utilize this published information as part of its NDA. Thus, it does not need to spend millions of dollars in discovering the drug, in doing biologic and toxicologic studies, and in conducting clinical trials. It can do a minimal amount of work to devise its own dosage forms, to establish stability, and to work out production and quality control procedures. A minimal amount of clinical investigation, designed only to show that the dosage form it intends to market behaves in humans as the original product does, will suffice. Thus, the cost of development will be, perhaps, something on the order of a hundred thousand dollars rather than $7 million. The huge sums spent by the innovator company in introducing the new drug to practicing physicians need not be matched by the second company, either. Since the physician already is aware of the drug and probably has had some experience in using it, it is necessary only to let him know of its availability (at a lower price) from the second supplier.

The situation in the future may become even more favorable for a second marketing company if patents covering drugs are abolished or severely limited in time, and if the view of former Commissioner James L. Goddard and some members of Congress prevails. In testimony before the Monopoly Subcommittee of the Senate Select Small Business Committee in 1967, Dr. Goddard suggested that Congress undertake a comprehensive review of the policy that data submitted by one firm cannot be made use of by another firm wishing to market the drug. He complained that the present policy "is wasteful of scientific talent." He went on to say: "We recognize that such a change raises questions about the circumstances under which data purchased with private money shall be placed in the public domain. But we also realize that the scientific community may have a valid need to know the detailed scientific basis for approval of a new drug that may be used by millions of people." In reply to a question from Senator Hugh Scott, Dr. Goddard conceded that "theoretically" such a change in policy would in effect subsidize companies that do not do extensive research of their own. However, he went on to state that he did not think this would change significantly the role of research-oriented pharmaceutical companies. "I think they would continue to be the main producers of new drug products," he said. "I don't think the situation would change."

I, for one, heartily disagree with a part of this conclusion. Research-oriented companies probably would remain the major source of new drug entities, but the rate of discovery and development of them probably would decrease drastically.

Some people also have argued that patents tend to limit further discoveries in the area covered by the patent. This certainly is not true for patents covering new drugs: when an important new patented drug appears, competitive firms immediately search for related drugs that are not covered by the original patent, but that can be covered by new patents, and usually some of these searches are successful and new drugs thus appear on the market. Often the new compounds have advantages over the earlier one; for example, they may be more potent, so that the dosage required is less than that of the original drug. Since the patient ingests less compound as a result of the lower dose, some of the side effects produced by the first drug may not appear; however, the increased potency

Patricia the collie over a 15-year period contributed to the research program that resulted in Diuril (MS&D). In 1959, she received from the National Society of Medical Research, as part of its Research Dog Hero of the Year program, the chain and locket shown here, and from the hands of Arlene Francis, the Special Today Award. (MS&D)

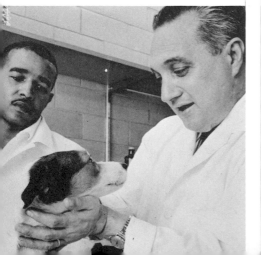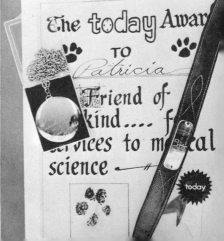

sometimes may cause the appearance of new side effects. In any case, the physician is presented with a choice of effective drugs. No two patients are alike biologically, and it may well turn out that one particular drug in a series is most useful for one patient, whereas another member works best for a second patient.

The research program that led to the discovery and marketing of chlorothiazide (Diuril, Merck Sharp & Dohme) was initiated about 14 years before the drug was marketed. This drug is used as a diuretic (agent to remove excessive fluid from the tissues) and in the treatment of high blood pressure. It was obvious to the entire industry that it was an important new drug, both medically and commercially. Within a few years, a number of related compounds not covered by the chlorothiazide patent appeared on the market. Some of them are listed in the following table.

GENERIC NAME	TRADEMARK & COMPANY	RANGE OF DAILY DOSAGE
Chlorothiazide	*Diuril* MS&D *	500-2,000 mg
Benzthiazide	*Aquatag* Tutag	50-150 mg
	Exna Robins	
Hydroflumethiazide	*Saluron* Bristol	25-200 mg
Hydrochlorothiazide	*HydroDiuril* MS&D *	50-100 mg
	Esidrix Ciba	
	Oretic Abbott	
Bendroflumethiazide	*Naturetin* Squibb	2-20 mg
Methylchlothiazide	*Induron* Abbott	2.5-15 mg
Bendromethiazide	*Benuron* Bristol	2.5-10 mg
Trichlormethiazide	*Metahydrin* Lakeside	2-8 mg
	Naqua Squibb	
Cyclothiazide	*Anhydron* Lilly	2-6 mg
Polythiazide	*Renese* Pfizer	1-4 mg

* Merck Sharp & Dohme.
mg = milligrams

Obviously, then, the introduction of the patented compound *chlorothiazide* to the market did not stifle research in its field.

Instead, it stimulated what amounts to a massive research effort that led to the introduction of an impressive list of effective compounds. The physician and his patients thus have a wide choice of therapeutic agents; if one of them is not sufficiently effective for a given patient, then a more useful related drug may be selected.

From time to time, there are proposals in the Congress to shorten the effective life of drug patents, which now are valid for 17 years after the patent is issued. Sometimes the proposals have been to require licensing of the patented drug to other companies at royalties with a stated maximum. Actually, the period of 17 years already has been shortened, at least insofar as the marketed drug is concerned, by the long period of time between discovery and actual marketing. Drug patents today usually issue from three to five years before marketing occurs, and thus the 17 years is reduced to 12 to 14 years.

Several years ago the eminent scientist, Dr. Vannevar Bush, testified before a Congressional committee considering modification of the patent system as it applies to drugs. Dr. Bush is Honorary Chairman and Life Member of the Corporation, Massachusetts Institute of Technology, has served as Chairman of the Board of Merck & Company, and was Director of the Office of Scientific Research and Development during World War II. He stated:

> I continue to be convinced, however, that the patent system is an essential part of our free enterprise system; that it has been responsible for a significant part of the great technical and industrial advance of this country; that in particular it has made possible the salutary advent of many small independent individual companies. . . .
>
> As far as patents are concerned, the central feature of the present bill is that it would require the licensing of all drug patents to all comers after a 3-year interval, and at royalties with a stated maximum.

The simple fact is that, if this were the law of the land, we would soon no longer lead the world in the development of new and useful drugs. Our industrial research programs on drug development would be severely cut back. How great a catastrophe this would be is not hard to visualize.

Only about three percent of the expenditures for research and development in the ethical pharmaceutical industry come from government grants or contracts. One reason for the reluctance of the Industry to accept such financial assistance is the probable loss of exclusive patent protection for a new product when all or a part of the expense of discovery and development has been financed by the government. According to government patent policy:

> Where . . . a principal purpose of the contract is for exploration into fields which directly concern the public health or public welfare . . . the government shall normally acquire or reserve the right to acquire the principal or exclusive rights throughout the world in and to any inventions made in the course of or under the contract. In exceptional cases the contractor may acquire greater rights than a non-exclusive license at the time of contracting, where the head of the department or agency certifies that such action will best serve the public interest. Greater rights may also be acquired by the contractor after the invention has been identified, where the invention when made in the course of or under the contract is not a primary object of the contract, provided the acquisition of such greater right is consistent with the intent of this Section . . . and is a necessary incentive to call forth private risk capital and expense to bring the invention to the point of practical application.

In 1965, President Johnson appointed a Commission to review the patent system. He stated that the present system was in need of reform because it takes much too long to receive a patent; the inventor frequently requires costly, time-consuming legal action to enforce his rights; the expense of obtaining a patent is too high; technological advances do not benefit the public quickly enough; and international trade is hindered by inconsistent patent practices between countries. In February, 1967, President Johnson sent the Patent Reform Act, based on the report of his Commission, to Congress. It has since been the subject of hearings in House and Senate committees.

Several provisions of this proposed act have been objectionable to many of those in the scientific and patent communities. The most controversial proposal is that the patent be granted to the first inventor to file in the Patent Office rather than to the first to make the invention. This would eliminate the possibility of interferences and would bring the United States system into line with that of the majority of other countries. Of the 74 countries that cooperate in the patent field, only three—the United States, Canada, and the Philippines—base priority on the "first to invent" system. Other controversial proposals include the elimination of the one year after publication, public use, or marketing grace period for filing the patent; automatic publication of pending patents (they are published now only after they have issued); and the mandatory rejection of patents covering computer programming.

The possibility of an international patent treaty is under study by six nations—France, Germany, Great Britain, Japan, the Soviet Union, and the United States. At present an inventor who seeks world-wide protection for his patent must make 74 applications in 20 languages; the treaty would provide for a single form that could be forwarded to all the countries in which the inventor wished to receive a patent. A patent search and examination would be carried out by one country, which would forward the results to all pertinent nations. Each country then would decide whether to issue a patent. Mr. Edward J. Brenner, then Commissioner of Patents, recently stated that 100,000 patent applications will be filed in the United States by 1970. Approximately 70,000 of these will be filed by US citizens and 30,000 by citizens of foreign countries. Of the 70,000 domestic-filed applications, approximately 30,000 will be filed in foreign countries. On the average, each of the 30,000 applications will be filed in 5 countries, so that about 150,000 foreign applications will be filed annually by US citizens. Of the more than half million patent applications filed annually throughout the world, approximately half are duplicate or multiple filings of the same invention.

TRADEMARKS

On February 20, 1905, an act authorizing the registration of trademarks used in interstate commerce (as well as in commerce with foreign nations and with the Indian tribes) became law. A trademark is defined as "a word, name, symbol, or device, or any combination of these, adopted and used by a manufacturer or merchant to indicate to purchasers that the quality of the goods bearing the mark remain constant, and it serves as the focal point of advertising disseminated to create and maintain a demand for the product." A trademark may be owned by an individual, a partnership or firm, a corporation, or an association or other collective group. Rights in a trademark are established by actual use of the mark on goods moving across state lines in trade. Ordinarily, the mark will remain the property of the user only if its use is continued. After goods bearing a trademark have been sold or shipped in interstate, foreign, or territorial commerce, the mark may be registered in the United States Patent Office. Even if it is not so registered, the trademark is protected under common law. A trademark may not be registered if it so resembles a mark previously registered in the Patent Office or previously used in the United States and not abandoned, as to be likely, when applied to the applicant's goods, to cause deception, mistake, or confusion. Marks that include the flag or insignia of the United States and marks that include immoral or deceptive matter cannot be registered.

The term of registration of a trademark is 20 years from the date of issue. It may be renewed at the end of each 20-year term so long as it still is in use in commerce.

COPYRIGHTS

Sometimes it is desirable for a research organization, or some member of it, to obtain a copyright. The scientific papers published by the research staff usually are copyrighted by their publishers. However, copyright protection may be desired for such things as brochures, periodicals, motion pictures, photographs, lectures, or drawing or plastic works of a scientific or technical character. Statutory copyrights may be obtained prior to publication for lectures, photographs, motion pictures other than photoplays, and musical compositions, but not for books or periodicals. Certificates of copyright are issued by the Register of Copyrights, in the Copyright Office, a branch of the Library of Congress. For lectures, photographs, and musical compositions, one complete copy must accompany the application for copyright. If the article is a motion picture other than a photoplay, then a title and description, together with at least two prints taken from different sections, must be sent to the Copyright Office.

An unpublished literary work, such as a research brochure,

is protected by "common law" copyright prior to publication. This type of protection is lost when the brochure is published and distributed. If the published brochure includes a correct notice of copyright inserted in the proper location, it then is protected by statutory copyright. This is true even if the copyright is not registered in the Copyright Office. However, the owner of the copyright cannot go into court to protect his right against infringement until the copyright is registered.

The copyright notice to be incorporated in the brochure or other article to be copyrighted must include the word "Copyright", the abbreviation "Copr.", or the symbol "©", accompanied by the name of the copyright owner and the year of first publication. In order to provide protection in all foreign countries that have ratified the Universal Copyright Convention, the notice should be given as follows:

Copyright © 1970 by (owner)
All Rights Reserved

In the case of a brochure, the copyright notice should appear upon the title page or the page immediately following. If the publication is a periodical, the notice may be placed either on the title page, or the first page of the text, or under the title heading. Two copies of books or periodicals must be sent to the Copyright Office after copyright has been secured by publication in order to obtain certification. A registered copyright is valid for 28 years. It may be renewed for a second 28-year period.

A statutory copyright is designed to grant to its owner a complete monopoly with respect to the copyrighted work. It allows him alone to reproduce and sell copies of the work in any form, and the adaptation and use of the work in any medium. It cannot be translated, broadcast, dramatized, published, or reproduced in any other way without the consent of the owner. There is one exception to this monopoly. This is the use permitted under the doctrine of "fair use." Thus a scholar or scientist is permitted to quote from and use scholarly and scientific works as a foundation for further contributions to knowledge. Also a criticism or review of a literary or artistic work may contain quotations required to make the criticism or review understandable.

CHAPTER 10

The Research Program

The Problems of Selection.
Available Areas

W HEN A RESEARCH DIRECTOR moves from one research group to head the research group in another company, he is confronted with several difficult problems. His ability to solve them smoothly, and without causing a major loss of morale in the research group, is a measure of his skill as a research administrator. He must be adept, too, at communicating his plans and objectives to top company management, and he must be effective in "selling" his ideas about the research program and its progress to management.

Chapters 1 and 2 have shown that a relatively large number of research skills are possessed by the scientists in a pharmaceutical research organization. In some industrial research and development laboratories, where almost all of the scientists are, for example, engineers or chemists, it is possible to transfer personnel from one research project to another with relative ease. This is hardly true in the pharmaceutical industry. Obviously, if increased manpower is required in the synthetic organic chemistry group, the problem cannot be solved by transferring microbiologists to the group. Similarly, organic chemists cannot be used to supplement the pathology group. In other words, the research program must, within limits, be built around the scientific skills and manpower available.

The only alternative to this is for the new research director to fire scientists whose skills are not required in his proposed

169

new program, and to hire replacements with the needed training and experience. Unquestionably, however, this is dangerous, and when it occurs, the inevitable result is that a number of the better scientists lose confidence in research management and seek, usually with success, jobs with competitive organizations. It becomes difficult, also, to interest good scientists in universities or other organizations in joining a research group whose management has shown its willingness to undertake wholesale firings, either for budgetary reasons or to change the direction of the research program. (I should perhaps hasten to state that when a scientist is fired for cause—incompetence, incompatible personality, immorality, and so on—his dismissal does not cause a morale problem.)

Most commonly, then, the research director will attempt to devise the best program possible with the skills available. As time passes, and scientists leave the organization, they can be replaced by others with new skills, and thus the program gradually can be modified as desirable. From a practical point of view, the scientists with the lowest turnover rate are mainly those with the doctor's degree. An appreciable number of scientists at the bachelor's degree level tend to leave the organization after a few years; many of these are young married women who work to help out during their first years of marriage, after which they leave to have families; the more capable younger men leave in order to take advanced degrees.

When budgets must be cut, almost always because of declining sales or profits of the parent organization, the research director usually resists suggestions from "across the street" that he do this by wholesale firing. Instead, commonly he institutes a policy of not rehiring when people leave the organization. Also—and this is unfortunate—usually he will curtail spending on projects done by scientists and clinicians outside his organization. Often curtailment involves a major decrease in the funds available for the clinical evaluation of potential new drugs: obviously this will decrease the rate of emergence of new products, but so will the alternative of firing large numbers of scientists. If the budget must be reduced drastically, there is no way to avoid a loss of productivity of the research group.

Another problem presented to every research director, new or old, in the pharmaceutical industry is that of attempting to establish a proper balance between the number of chemists who are synthesizing potential new drugs and the number of biologists who are testing them for biologic activity. As each budget period approaches, the biologists point out that they do not have sufficient manpower to test all of the new compounds presented in all of the biologic tests available. Therefore, they argue, why hire more chemists, who will make still more compounds and thus "compound" the problem? Why not, instead, hire more biologists in order to approach the ideal goal of testing all new compounds in all available tests? After all, a valuable new drug may be sitting on some chemist's shelf, unrecognized because it has not been tested. The chemists quickly point out that usually new compounds are made as members of a chemical series, and almost always at least some members of the series are widely tested; presumably, other members of the series will have similar biologic properties. If additional chemists become available, the variety of different types of chemical compound available for testing will be greater, and this, say the chemists, should increase the possibility of finding a valuable new drug.

Each research director must arrive at a solution of this problem in his own way. Some have suggested that research directors with chemical backgrounds favor the chemists' point of view, whereas those who were trained in biology or biochemistry tend to support the biologists. From my own observations over the years, I think there is at least some truth to this. As to which solution is *right*—more chemists or more biologists—well, there just is no answer to that question.

❧ ❧

A very few large pharmaceutical research organizations have sufficient manpower to undertake research in almost every branch of experimental therapeutics. In most cases, however, the research director must conclude that limitations of manpower and research funds require that only certain fields can be investigated. How does he decide what these fields will be? He has certain broad guidelines. For one thing, his company might have made decisions that are helpful; management might have decided, for example, that it does not wish to enter biologics, that to do so might involve large capital outlays to construct proper production facilities. Sometimes the detail force is well trained in certain types of therapeutic agents that are profitable to the company, and management indicates its interest in strengthening the company position in these fields. Often, however, the research director's judgment also is desired by management, and usually he presents his proposed program to management at least annually.

Another guideline is furnished by a listing of the types of therapeutic agent available and a breakdown of their sales. This gives an indication of the probable commercial importance of each type. The following table, using figures compiled by Arthur D. Little, Inc., lists the sales of different groups of ethical drugs in 1967.

THERAPEUTIC GROUP	MANUFACTURERS' SELLING PRICES, 1967, IN MILLIONS OF DOLLARS
Antibiotics	$ 470
Ataraxics (tranquilizers)	310
Hormones (including oral contraceptive drugs)	298
Vitamins and nutrients	220
Cardiovascular drugs	200
Analgesics	150
Cough and cold preparations	120
Diabetes mellitus therapy	94
Diuretics	92
Antiobesity	86
Antispasmodics	68
Sedatives	67
Antiarthritics	65
Antacids	62
Sulfonamides	50
Psychostimulants	44
Hematinics (drugs for anemia)	40
Antihistamines	38
Muscle relaxants	35
Others	830
Total Ethical Sales	*$3,339*

Another useful guideline is furnished by an examination of the major causes of death in the United States. The following table, compiled from information published by the Department of Health, Education, and Welfare, lists some of these.

CAUSES OF DEATH		NUMBER OF DEATHS 1965
Cardiovascular-renal disease		1,002,112
Coronary disease	559,293	
Strokes	201,057	
High blood pressure	66,635	
Cancer		297,588
Infectious diseases		165,647
Accidents		108,004
Motor vehicles	49,163	
Accidents in the home	24,086	
Others	34,755	
Diabetes mellitus		33,174
Cirrhosis of the liver		24,715
Senility and other ill-defined conditions		23,414
Suicide		20,588
Congenital malformations		19,512
Homicides		10,712
Asthma		4,520
Enlargement of the prostate gland		3,412
Complications of childbirth		1,189
All other causes		92,202

◆§ §◆

Diseases of the heart and blood vessels (often with secondary involvement of the kidneys) claim the lives of more than 1,000,000 Americans each year. This is more than all other causes of death combined. It is not surprising, then, that almost all pharmaceutical research groups have programs in this area of disease. The greatest number of these deaths are caused by disease of the coronary vessels, the blood vessels that carry food and oxygen to, and carbon dioxide and waste products away from, the heart muscle. The most common disease is atherosclerosis, a condition in which deposits of fatty materials (including cholesterol) form in and on the inner layers of the arteries in the body, including the coronary arteries. The risk of coronary disease is highest in obese males who smoke cigarettes and who have high blood cholesterol levels and blood pressures. The death rate from all forms of cardiovascular disease, including coronary disease, is lower in women than in men; this feminine advantage is most marked between the ages of 25 and 64. The American Heart Association has estimated that 3,125,000 of the 14,621,000 Americans who have definite heart disease have coronary disease. An additional 6,900,000 Americans have definite high blood pressure without heart disease, and heart disease is suspected, but not proved, in 12,979,000 additional cases.

Unfortunately, it is difficult to use experimental coronary disease as a screening procedure in the research laboratory. This type of disease, including death from coronary occlusion, can be produced in animals, although it is not certain that the experimental disease is identical with the human disorder. In one procedure, for example, one kidney is removed from a rat and a ligature is tied around the remaining kidney; animals so treated develop a persistent high blood pressure. The treated animals then are fed only ground beef, salts, vitamins, and water. Half the calories of ground beef come from animal fat. In something like 15 weeks most of the animals exhibit elevated levels of cholesterol, fats, and fat-like substances in the blood; at about 30 weeks, many of them have well-developed atherosclerosis of the coronary arteries, and some of these animals actually die of coronary occlusion.

The long period of time required to produce the disorder makes it impossible to screen large numbers of new compounds as potential agents to prevent or cure the coronary disease in these rats. Actually, so far as I am aware, the only drugs that have been proved effective agents are drugs that lower blood pressure. No drug that will reverse the established disease has been found. Many long-term statistical studies in humans have indicated that individuals who have a high level of cholesterol in the blood have an increased chance of developing significant atherosclerosis—and thus an increased risk of coronary disease and strokes. According to the American Heart Association, a man with a cholesterol level of 260 mg (milligrams) per 100 ml (milliliters) of plasma (the liquid portion of the blood) runs more than three times the risk of a heart attack than the man whose plasma cholesterol is below 200 mg per 100 ml.

It is understandable, then, that pharmaceutical research laboratories would search for new drugs that will lower the level of cholesterol in the plasma. The drug, triparanol, was marketed by the William S. Merrell Company under their trademark, MER-29, in 1959. Although this compound was quite effective in lowering plasma cholesterol, it produced such severe toxicity in some patients that it was removed from the market in April, 1962. I am sure that this unfortunate experience caused some research laboratories to abandon their interest in this field. However, others persisted, and two new drugs that are effective in lowering plasma cholesterol levels appeared on the market in 1967. They are clofibrate (Atromid-S, Ayerst) and sodium dextrothyroxine (Choloxin, Flint). Atromid-S decreases the synthesis of cholesterol in the liver. The rationale for the development of Choloxin is interesting: when the thyroid gland secretes too much hormone (hyperthyroidism), the level of plasma cholesterol falls; when too little hormone is secreted (hypothyroidism), the level rises. Now Choloxin has exactly the same chemical structure as L-thyroxine, one of the hormones of the thyroid gland, except that some of the atoms in its molecule have a different arrangement in space. This slight change causes the drug to be much less active than thyroxine in producing the hormonal activities of the thyroid gland. However, it retains the property of reducing the level of plasma cholesterol. Probably it will be a number of years before it can be decided whether this type of drug will reduce the number of coronary attacks and strokes. In the meantime, undoubtedly other companies will market new drugs in this area.

It has been demonstrated experimentally that the plasma level of cholesterol can be lowered in human subjects if a substantial part of the animal fat in their diets is replaced by vegetable fat. However, ingesting capsules of vegetable fat without a substantial reduction in the intake of animal fat has no effect on the level of cholesterol in the blood.

An appreciable number of patients with coronary atherosclerosis have a condition known as *angina pectoris*. These are Latin words: *angina* means "to strangle" or, sometimes, "distress," and *pectoris* means "of the breast." Angina pectoris is characterized by sudden attacks of pain felt beneath the sternum (breastbone). Usually it is of short duration, but it is frightening since it causes a sense of apprehension or even fear of impending death. An attack most commonly is precipitated by an emotional upset or by physical exertion. It can be relieved by rest and by allowing a small tablet of nitroglycerin to dissolve under the tongue. The attack is caused by an increase in the work done by the heart because of the emotional or physical stress. When this occurs, the narrowed coronary vessels cannot transport enough oxygen and food to, and enough carbon dioxide and waste products away from, the cells of the heart muscle, and this results in the pain experienced by the patient. Unfortunately, animals seldom tell us when they have pain, and, if angina pectoris ever occurs in them, we cannot recognize it. However, several drugs that are useful in preventing, or at least in decreasing the frequency of, attacks of angina pectoris in man are on the market. A number of studies designed to learn how these drugs act on the heart are going on in pharmaceutical research laboratories, and from such studies have emerged several tests for this type of activity. Hopefully, these tests will permit the discovery of more effective drugs in the future.

High blood pressure can be produced in experimental animals by several procedures; the commonest, perhaps, is the method already described earlier in this chapter. Probably it is true that hypertension (high blood pressure) in humans may have several causes: in most cases, we do not really know the cause, and so compounds usually are screened in the laboratory on a "hit or miss" basis. This type of screening has resulted in the discovery and marketing of a number of drugs useful in lowering blood pressure; none of them really cures the disorder, although some patients who have been treated with certain of them for many years can stop taking them without a return of their hypertension. In a few cases, the cause of the hypertension may be a small tumor in the adrenal gland or a constriction in the artery entering the kidney. These often can be cured by surgery.

In heart disease of long duration, the condition known as congestive heart failure may occur. In this condition, the heart is enlarged and does not have the strength to pump sufficient blood throughout the body, which results in shortness of breath (cardiac asthma) on exertion, accumulation of large amounts of water and salt in the extremities, abdomen, and tissues (edema), and weakness. For many years, digitalis and compounds isolated from it have been the drugs used to stimulate and strengthen such a heart. Unfortunately, the toxic dose of digitalis is very close to the therapeutic dose, and there is great need for a better drug, for which many laboratories are searching.

Often the immediate cause of death in heart disease is cardiac arrhythmia. Normally, of course, the heart beats rhythmically, pumping out blood in systole (contraction of heart muscles) and filling with blood in diastole (relaxation of heart muscles). In an arrhythmia (there are different types), the contractions of the heart muscles become very rapid and often occur in different parts of the heart at different times. Sometimes there is a blockade, so that some portions of the heart have no or infrequent contractions. If this condition persists very long, the patient will die, since the arrhythmic heart cannot pump blood through the body in adequate amounts. Only two drugs are available as therapeutic agents for this cardiac complication. One is an old natural drug, quinidine, the other a newer synthetic one—procainamide hydrochloride (Pronestyl, Squibb). Physical instruments, such as electrical defibrillators and pacemakers, may cause the heart rhythm to revert to normal, and have proved lifesaving in many cases. Various operative procedures for producing experimental cardiac arrhythmias in animals are available. A number of research laboratories have programs designed to find more effective drugs in this area.

One type of drug that is of major therapeutic importance in cardiovascular disease is the modern diuretic. The word *modern* is used because, although diuretics have been available for many years, they were of sharply limited value compared to the agents that have appeared since 1958. In that year, Merck Sharp & Dohme introduced chlorothiazide under their trademark, Diuril. This drug increases the excretion of sodium, chiefly in the form of sodium chloride (table salt) in the urine. Since the salt is dissolved in water, the excretion of water also is enhanced. This type of drug is useful in increasing the loss of salt and water from the body in conditions under which these substances accumulate in excessive amounts in the tissues. (This excess storage of salty fluid is termed *edema;* an older term is *dropsy.*) Usually this occurs in diseases of the kidneys, liver, and, perhaps most commonly, the heart (congestive heart failure).

It had been known before the availability of Diuril that restriction of salt in the diet was of value in lowering the blood pressure in hypertension. It is not surprising, then that chlorothiazide and related drugs also are extremely valuable in the management of hypertension. Commonly they are given to the patient along with a second drug that lowers blood pressure by a different mechanism. The story of the discovery of chlorothiazide is related in Chapter 2. Some diuretics of similar chemical structures are listed in a table in Chapter 9.

ومج وبه

The second largest killer of Americans is cancer: almost 300,000 deaths were caused by this type of disease in 1965. The American Cancer Society estimates that 600,000 new cases of cancer were found in 1968. Probably one of every four living Americans will suffer from cancer, and two of every three families will be affected. In spite of the obvious importance of cancer as a medical problem, only a few pharmaceutical research laboratories have research programs in this area. One chief reason is that we simply do not have leads that give a rational basis for the synthesis and screening of potential drugs in this field. Of course, a number of drugs are used in therapy; a few are hormones, or compounds with hormonal activity—ordinarily given in dosages sufficiently high to cause toxicity if used too long—but most of them are cell poisons that exert their greatest toxicity on young, multiplying cells. When they are used, the hope is that they can be given in a dosage that will cause the death of the cancer cells (which are young and rapidly multiplying) without doing too much damage to normal tissue cells. In other words, they really are not specific for cancer. As a matter of fact, the term *cancer* embraces a large number of malignant diseases, and if and when a cure for one type of cancer is found, it may well be ineffective for other types.

We must, then, resort to random screening of compounds and potential antibiotic broths against selected animal cancers as a method of searching for an effective agent. Now, a number of laboratories supported by governmental funds will do this, and most pharmaceutical research groups send selected compounds and microbial broths to them for screening. This program has been a massive one; more than $1 billion of governmental money has gone into it. Pharmaceutical firms have contributed a great deal of time and effort in cooperating with the government; in addition to donating most of the substances screened, these companies have furnished the advisory services of a group of their research directors. Unfortunately, this huge project, as well as similar screening programs at several cancer institutes, has not produced therapeutic agents specific for cancer.

◄§ §►

Infectious diseases caused the death of 165,647 Americans in 1965 and, from an economic point of view, are the most important group of diseases. The greatest loss of time from work is caused by the common cold, which does not kill, but which attacks many times during a lifetime. The annual sales of drugs used in the treatment of infections (antibiotics, sulfonamides, cough and cold preparations) totaled $640 million at manufacturers' selling prices in 1967.

For bacterial infections, it is rather easy to establish a screening program that is rapid enough to permit the testing of all the new compounds made by the chemists. Selected pathogenic bacteria are grown in test tubes, and the compounds then are added to these tubes. If bacterial growth is stopped, the test is repeated, except that this time some animal serum (the fluid that oozes from a blood clot) also is added to the tubes. Many compounds that were active in the first test are inactivated by the serum—an indication that they probably would not be active in the body. If a compound is active even in the presence of serum, it is tested against an actual infection, usually in mice. If it either prevents or cures the disease in the animals (a rare event), it becomes a candidate to be worked up for possible clinical testing.

ᴇᴷ ᴀᴇ

Some laboratories have active programs in antibiotics, a complicated field of research; not very many truly important antibiotics have been discovered in recent years. The usual procedure is to obtain samples of soil from almost anywhere, sometimes from many parts of the world. Thousands of such samples are tested annually. The samples are mixed with a broth medium in which microorganisms in the soil will grow. (Most marketed antibiotics have been found in a group of soil microorganisms known as *actinomycetes*.) Samples of material from these growing cultures then are added to test tubes in which various types of pathogenic organisms are growing, and if the sample is active, that is, inhibits the growth of the test organisms, the real work begins.

At this point, it is necessary to find out whether the active ingredient made by the soil microorganism is a new antibiotic or one that has been discovered earlier. In some programs, as many as 1 in 5 soil samples tested have yielded an antibiotic, but in most cases it was not new; one fairly small antibiotic research group, for example, found oxytetracycline 200 times in a single year. Sometimes scientists can determine whether the antibiotic is new or old with the aid of bacteria that have been "trained" to be resistant to one or more of the known antibiotics. In other cases, sufficient material to permit chemists to isolate and purify the active material must be grown in culture medium, so that the pure material then can be compared directly with known purified antibiotics.

If the antibiotic is new, the next problem is to prepare enough of it to determine its toxicity in animals. Most new antibiotics, unfortunately, are highly toxic. Finally, if toxicity is not too high, animals infected with representative disease-producing organisms are treated with the new antibiotic. Often the new agent is not effective in this test. If it *is* effective, then, of course, it must be worked up by the pharmacologists, microbiologists, biochemists, toxicologists, and pathologists to determine whether it can safely be tested in humans. It is my own personal opinion that laboratories that do not already have an active antibiotic program probably should not initiate one. The number of scientists required is rather large and the odds of success are rather low.

◆§ ဦ◆

For many years, scientists have searched for a drug that would be effective against infections caused by viruses. Compounds (or cultures) can be screened *in vitro* (that is, by adding them to the culture fluids in which cells infected with viruses are growing in tissue culture) on *in vivo*. In the latter type of screen, usually the experimental compound is given to animals (most commonly, mice), after which amounts of various viruses capable of producing a fatal infection are administered. An effective material should prevent death caused by the viral infection. Only a few interesting compounds have emerged from these years of searching, and only two drugs in the area are marketed in the United States. One is idoxuridine (Stoxil, Smith Kline & French; Dendrid, Alcon Laboratories; Herplex, Allergan Pharmaceuticals); it is used topically in the treatment of herpes simplex keratitis, a superficial (surface) infection of the cornea (the transparent portion of the eye). The lesion is branched like the veins in a leaf, with knoblike terminals, and a hazard to vision, since untreated cases tend to recur with the formation of ulcers and opaque scars. Fortunately, the disease is rare, and most cases respond favorably to treatment with idoxuridine.

E. I. du Pont de Nemours & Company have entered the pharmaceutical field by marketing the antiviral drug, amantadine hydrochloride, under their trademark, Symmetrel. The only substantiated use for this drug is in the prophylaxis (prevention) of infection caused by a specific strain of influenza virus (type A_2, also known as the Asian strain). The drug will not cure the disease after it is established in a patient, but is most useful in helping to prevent infection in those who must be in close contact with a patient infected with type A_2 influenza virus. It may be used also in people who are especially susceptible to infection with influenza virus, particularly when cases of infection due to type A_2 have been reported in the neighborhood. Such people are often those suffering from chronic, debilitating diseases (such as those of the cardiovascular system, lungs, and kidneys), and persons in the older age group.

A compound known as beta-thiosemicarbazone has been reported effective in suppressing infection caused by smallpox virus even after exposure to the virus has occurred. The clinical trial of this compound, which originated in England, was carried out in India. If we ever are so fortunate as to discover a chemotherapeutic agent that is effective against a wide variety of viral diseases, it may be useful also in treating cancer. A number of animal cancers are known to be caused by viruses.

Many scientists suspect that at least some types of cancer in humans are initiated by viruses. Several companies that market biologics have become interested in the development and manufacture of viral vaccines. One reason for entering the field was the hope that a vaccine effective in preventing the common cold could be found. This hope has all but vanished, however. Several hundred viruses capable of causing upper respiratory infections have been discovered, and undoubtedly many more will be. Since they do not give cross immunity (that is, a vaccine prepared from one of them will not protect against the others), an effective vaccine would have to contain antigens from hundreds—perhaps thousands—of different viruses. One prominent virologist pointed out some years ago that it is *possible* that every cold a person has during his lifetime is caused by a different virus. Perhaps this explains why we do not become immune to colds.

Parainfluenza (types 1, 2, and 3) and the respiratory syncytial (RS) viruses are important causative agents of viral pneumonia and upper respiratory infections in children. *Mycoplasma pneumoniae*, formerly known as the Eaton agent, causes viral pneumonia in both children and adults. Adenoviruses (types 1, 2, 3, 5, and 6) cause respiratory illness in children, also, and adenoviruses (types 3, 4, 7, 14, and 21) have been the cause of epidemics in military recruits. The military used an effective adenovirus vaccine for several years, but its use was stopped when it was found that types 3, 7, 12, 14, 16, 18, 21 and 31 caused cancer when injected into hamsters.

Rhinoviruses probably are the major cause of the common cold in adults; they also cause colds and pneumonia in children. In a talk given in 1966, Dr. Maurice R. Hilleman, who directs the research program in virology and cell biology in the Merck Institute for Therapeutic Research, stated: "The principal problem from the vaccine standpoint is that of extreme diversity of distinct serotypes" (of rhinoviruses). "Fifty-three numbered serotypes have been established and the total probably numbers into the hundreds or even thousands."

Viral vaccines developed in recent years have been extremely important medically. The Salk and Sabin vaccines have all but wiped out poliomyelitis in this country. Only 16 cases of acute poliomyelitis were reported in the United States in 1965. Measles (rubeola) vaccine, has decreased markedly the incidence of measles. Live attenuated measles vaccine was marketed in the United States in 1963. During 1967, the number of reported cases in this country declined to less than 13 percent of the average number reported annually before the vaccine was available. The National Communicable Disease Center in Atlanta predicts that this figure will decline to 5 percent in 1968. The actual number of new cases forecast for 1968 was only 15,000 to 20,000. This same experience can be predicted for mumps if the new vaccine, marketed early in 1968 by Merck Sharp & Dohme, proves as safe and effective as it appeared to be during clinical testing. The mildness of mumps in children may limit its use, however.

On the other hand, these modern vaccines have not been too rewarding commercially. I suspect that the several companies that developed the Salk vaccine all eventually actually lost money on the product. The Sabin vaccine is so potent that only tiny doses are required, and I can't imagine that the sales figures for this product can be very large. With measles vaccine, there is a tendency for governmental health agencies, at several organizational levels, to purchase it as cheaply as possible and to make it available free or at nominal cost to children.

One viral vaccine that should be extremely valuable, both medically and commercially, is a vaccine against rubella (German measles). When pregnant women become ill with this infection during the first trimester (3 months) of pregnancy,

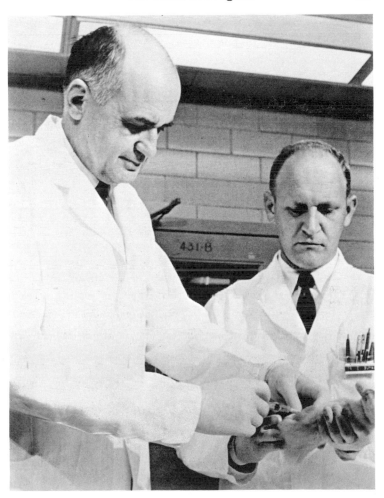

One safety test for the new rubella vaccine is performed here on a live young duckling by Drs. Maurice Hilleman and Eugene Buynak, who headed the MS&D Laboratories scientists developing the vaccine. (MS&D)

the incidence of congenital defects in their offspring increases markedly. Of the more than a dozen congenital defects that have been observed, the most common are heart disease, cataracts, deafness, and mental retardation. Since most affected adults contract the disease from children, it is desirable to vaccinate *all* young people who have not already had the disease. Every young woman is a potential candidate for vaccination unless she has antibodies against the disease in her bloodstream (indicating prior infection), or unless she is possibly or actually pregnant. The vaccine has not yet been tested in pregnant women; conceivably, it might itself cause congenital defects if administered to this group.

An epidemic of rubella occurred in the United States in 1963-1965, and in the fall of 1969, some 30,000 rubella-damaged children entered the first grade of school. It has been estimated that it will cost at least $4.8 billion to educate and care for these children. Live rubella virus vaccine was made available in the United States in June, 1969, by Merck Sharp & Dohme Laboratories, under its trademark, Lyovac Meruvax. At least three other United States firms (Philips Roxane Laboratories, Eli Lilly and Company, and Smith Kline & French Laboratories) are developing rubella virus vaccines.

The very first vaccine to become available to the medical profession was a viral vaccine. Edward Jenner (1749-1823), an English physician, found that when material obtained from the vesicles on the skin of cattle that had the disease known as cowpox (now usually known as vaccinia) was introduced into the skin of humans, they became immune to smallpox. Commercial smallpox vaccine (really live vaccinia virus) still is prepared as a glycerinated suspension of the fluid from the vesicles of vaccinia that have formed on the skin of healthy calves inoculated with vaccinia virus.

Influenza viral vaccine contains a mixture of known strains

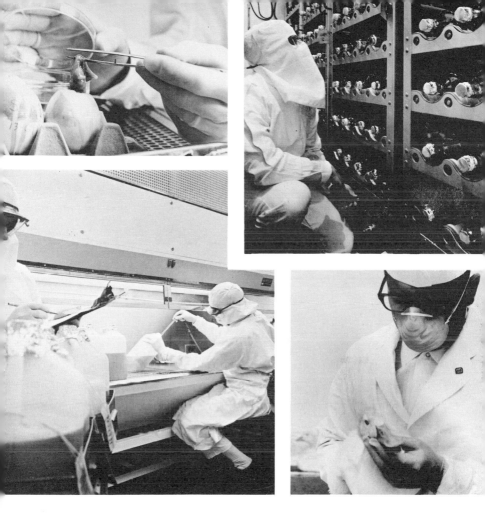

Embryos from fertilized eggs of Pekin ducks are used to produce the new German measles vaccine at the West Point, Pennsylvania, plant of MS&D. The attenuated virus is grown on sheets of duck cells formed on the rounded sides of bottles, rotated so that the cell sheets are continually bathed in a nutrient. Only the most sterile conditions are permitted—garments are sanitary, air filtered. Veterinarian D. Phelben is responsible for the welfare of the ducks, their swimming pool shown in the background. (MS&D)

of influenza virus. Each year a guessing game develops between the scientists and technicians who prepare this vaccine and nature. Most infection each year is caused by only one strain of the virus, but often this is a new strain that differs somewhat from those previously known. The trick is to incorporate this new "mutant" into the current vaccine. When this is done successfully, the vaccine is 75 to 95 percent effective. If world-wide surveillance is not effective enough to permit incorporation of the new strain, the vaccine may be rather ineffective. This was the situation in this country, for example, in 1967. Influenza virus protein is rather toxic, and some people who receive the vaccine, especially children, suffer a reaction. Some laboratories are attempting to prepare less toxic influenza vaccine. Other viral vaccines available include those used for protection against rabies, yellow fever, Western, Eastern, and Venezuelan encephalomyelitis, and Japanese encephalitis.

One defense the body has against viral infection is the production in infected cells of a substance known as *interferon*. This protein imparts a broad-spectrum resistance to viral infection in those body cells not yet infected by the virus. Interferon is species specific; that is, each animal species makes its own "private brand." It is not effective after the infection has become established, but when injected into animals before infection has become established, it can prevent clinical infection, being active in tiny amounts.

It does not appear feasible to isolate interferon and use it as a drug. For one thing, to be effective in humans, probably it would have to be isolated from human cells. Fortunately, however, animal experimentation indicates that it may prove feasible to stimulate the body to make its own interferon. Thus, certain natural substances have been found effective in stimulating the formation and release of interferon when they are injected into animals. A number of laboratories are searching for an effective stimulant suitable for use in clinical experimentation.

◦§ ◦

Mental illness, although not listed among the causes of death, certainly is a major cause of illness. Chlorpromazine hydrochloride (Thorazine, Smith Kline & French) was the first of the "major" tranquilizers to be marketed, and a number of drugs with similar therapeutic activity have been made available since. This type of agent has been of tremendous help in the treatment of the psychoses—that is, major mental diseases, such as schizophrenia, that involve a disintegration of the personality and its break with reality. These drugs are not curative, but they have been so effective in controlling the psychoses that many patients have adjusted well enough to live at home and even to work effectively. In 1955, the first widely used "minor" tranquilizer (meprobamate, discovered and marketed by Wallace Pharmaceuticals under their trademark, Miltown) became available, and was marketed at about the same time by Wyeth Laboratories, whose trademark was Equanil. Several other firms now market the drug, both as an entity and in combination dosage forms. This type of tranquilizer is not useful in the treatment of true psychoses, but is helpful in the management of common psychoneurotic conditions characterized by anxiety and nervous tension.

Serpasil, CIBA Pharmaceutical Company's trademark for reserpine, and some other drugs made from the Indian plant, *Rauwolfia serpentina*, were marketed in 1953. They are useful mainly in the treatment of hypertension, but have some activity also against mental disease.

Following the marketing of these useful agents, some research managements decided that new agents in this area would be highly competitive and probably not too interesting commercially. How wrong they were! Roche Laboratories made Librium (the Roche trademark for chlordiazepoxide HCl) available in 1960. It is classed as a "minor" tranquilizer, but it is more potent than meprobamate. Chlordiazepoxide and a related compound, diazepam (Valium, Roche) accounted for 38 percent of the total sales of tranquilizers in 1967 (chlordiazepoxide, 23 percent; diazepam, 15 percent). Diazepam is useful also as a muscle relaxant in patients with muscular spasm, such as children with cerebral palsy and adults who have recovered from strokes. Most pharmaceutical research laboratories have programs in the field of mental illness. In addition to better major and minor tranquilizers, they are searching for agents to treat mental depression that will be more effective than those now available.

◄§ §►

Many laboratories are searching for better drugs to control conception. (The oral tablets presently marketed in this area should be referred to as contraceptive rather than "birth-control" drugs. They are believed to act by the prevention of conception—that is, effective union of the egg and sperm—and not by an effect on the birth process itself.) After the age of puberty, the normal human female releases an ovum (egg) from one of her ovaries at about the middle of each menstrual cycle. Ova cease to be expelled after the menopause. Shortly before expulsion of the ovum occurs, it is located in a hollow space, called a follicle, in the ovary. At ovulation, this follicle breaks open at the surface of the ovary, and the ovum escapes into the body cavity. The ruptured follicle then fills with a blood clot, which is replaced in a few days by large cells that have a yellow color. This mass of cells is called the corpus luteum ("yelow body"). If pregnancy does not occur, the corpus luteum is replaced by scar tissue, but if the ovum is fertilized, the corpus luteum remains intact during the first few months of pregnancy.

Hormones made by the cells that line the follicles (as well as synthetic compounds with similar biologic properties) are known as *estrogens*. (These hormones are responsible for the periodic occurrence of estrus—desire on the part of the female for mating—in the lower animals.) They are responsible for the development of secondary sex characteristics at puberty—growth of the breasts, distribution of body hair, changes in the uterus and vagina. During a menstrual period, the lining of the uterus (the endometrium) largely sloughs off and is expelled with the menstrual blood; the regeneration of this lining that begins after menstruation is governed by the estrogenic hormones. At about the time of expulsion of the ovum (usually at about day 14 after the beginning of the menstrual period, but don't count on it!), the secretion of estrogen diminishes, and shortly after this the corpus luteum begins to secrete a second ovarian hormone, *progesterone*. This substance prepares the lining of the uterus for the nourishment and attachment of the fertilized ovum. If the ovum is not fertilized, the production of progesterone ceases rather abruptly on about day 23 or 24 of the menstrual cycle, and menstruation soon follows.

Now these events—the secretion of estrogens, ovulation, formation of the corpus luteum, secretion of progesterone, decrease in the secretion of both estrogens and progesterone during the menstrual cycle—are regulated by hormones that are manufactured by the anterior pituitary gland, a small structure located at the base of the brain. The contraceptive tablet first marketed contains a mixture of an estrogen and a progestogen (compound with biologic activity like the natural hormone, progesterone). One tablet is taken each day beginning on day 5 of the menstrual period and continuing for 20 days. A new series of 20 tablets is started on day 5 of the next menstrual period. The amount of estrogen in the tablets is sufficient to inhibit the secretion of some of the pituitary hormones and this prevents ovulation (expulsion of the egg from the ovary). Thus, no egg is released into the body cavity. Normally, ova that are released from the ovary travel down the Fallopian tube that leads from the vicinity of the ovary to the interior of the uterus. If the ovum is fertilized, this occurs by union of a spermatozoan with the ovum during its passage down the Fallopian tube. If no ovum is released, obviously conception cannot take place.

Now, the incorporation of the progestogen in the tablet is useful mainly in reassuring the woman that pregnancy has not occurred. Thus, a few days after she discontinues taking the tablets on the twentieth day, the abrupt withdrawal of the progestogen results in a sloughing of the lining of the uterus, a process identical with the menstrual period that occurs normally when the corpus luteum ceases to manufacture progesterone. This is a signal that pregnancy has not occurred. Since the progestogen really is not required during most of the interval between menstrual periods, the "sequential method" of administering estrogen and progestogen as contraceptive agents was developed. In this method, the woman takes tablets containing only an estrogen for 15 days, beginning on day 5 of the menstrual period. Then comes a mixture of estrogen and progestogen for the next 5 days. Menstruation usually begins a few days after the last tablet is taken. Medication from a new package then is started on day 5 of this menstrual period.

Other modifications are under investigation in the clinic. One experimental procedure involves the oral ingestion of a single tablet only once each 28 days. This tablet contains a long-acting estrogen and a progestogen whose activity persists for only a few days. The woman starts by taking one such tablet on the first, second, or third day of a menstrual period. The estrogen present is sufficiently potent and long-lasting to inhibit the pituitary gland, and ovulation thus does not occur during this cycle. The progestogen in this first tablet is not required, but is included for simplicity. An identical second tablet is taken 3 weeks later. This has two functions. The estrogen present will inhibit ovulation during the next 28 days; the progestogen will thicken the endometrium that has been stimulated to grow by the first dose of estrogen, but its effect will wear off in a short time. Menstruation then occurs in a few days. A tablet then is taken every 28 days so long as protection from conception is desired.

Another "once a month" method involves giving the combination of estrogen and progestogen by injection rather than by mouth. Usually this requires a visit to the doctor's office. Injectable contraceptive drugs designed to be effective for three to six months are being studied in the clinic. Apparently, also, conception can be prevented by giving the woman a small dose of progestogen every day, including the days of menstruation, and beginning on the first day of a menstrual period. This does not prevent menstruation, which normally occurs each 28 to 35 days or so. Just why this prevents conception is not known. The method is experimental at present. In a variation of this method, the woman takes a tablet of the progestogen within 12 hours after sexual intercourse, and not at other times. There has not been sufficient experience with this procedure to judge its probable effectiveness, although initial results are encouraging. One clinical report, summarizing an investigator's experience with this method, states, "Some patients have taken nearly 30 capsules per month with no complications other than exhaustion."

Research laboratories also are searching for drugs that will inhibit the union of the sperm and the egg; interfere with the passage of the sperm from the vagina to the Fallopian tube; and interfere with nidation (the implantation of a fertilized ovum in the lining of the uterus). Some research programs include a search for agents that would be taken by the male rather than by the female. This type of drug might act to inhibit the formation or functioning of the spermatazoa.

◄§ §►

Almost all pharmaceutical research organizations have a program designed to discover new analgesics (drugs that reduce or eliminate pain). Aspirin, an analgesic that anyone can purchase, of course, without a prescription, is the most widely used drug in existence today. In thinking about this problem, pharmacologists tend to classify analgesics as "aspirin-like" or "morphine-like." Aspirin is a weak analgesic as compared to morphine, but it has some real advantages. It is effective by mouth, it performs adequately when the pain is mild, it has some anti-inflammatory activity (and hence is useful in painful swellings and bruises, as well as in chronic inflammatory diseases such as arthritis), it is nonaddicting, and certainly it is cheap. Morphine, on the other hand, must be given by injection and carries the danger of addiction. It is effective, however, even against the severe pain that accompanies some cases of terminal cancer. Both aspirin and morphine can cause distressing side effects, but morphine is much more likely to cause them.

Since animals cannot tell us when they experience pain, there is often some doubt that screening procedures actually are measuring pain. This doubt is underlined by the fact that a number of compounds that have been active in the laboratory have not proved useful in the clinic. A major difficulty in developing a new analgesic is that of proving effectiveness in the clinic. In most controlled clinical studies, the placebo has relieved the pain in from 30 to 50 percent of the patients, morphine in about 85 percent of the patients. These figures are rather close to each other, and it is perhaps not surprising that analgesics weaker than morphine often do not show very well. In some trials, it has not been possible to differentiate the new drug, aspirin, codeine, and the placebo from each other. The ideal analgesic would be at least as potent as morphine but without the liability of addiction and the other side effects caused by morphine, and, also, active by mouth. Perhaps the closest approach to this ideal is exemplified by pentazocine, marketed by Winthrop Laboratories under their trademark, Talwin, an injected dose of 30 mg (milligrams) of which is about as effective as 10 mg of morphine. It is active both by injection and by mouth. It is free of some of the side effects of morphine: it does not cause addiction when it is given by mouth, and usually does not cause constipation, urinary retention, or severe respiratory depression (tendency on the part of the patient to breathe very slowly or even to stop breathing).

꠸꠸ ꠸꠸

The term, *hypersensitivity*, refers to a state in which the body, usually following exposure to an antigen, develops antibodies or, perhaps, sensitized cells that act like antibodies. When these antibodies or sensitized cells encounter, and react with, the antigen, a reaction occurs. Sometimes this reaction is favorable and sometimes it is harmful. Antigens capable of stimulating the formation of antibodies usually are proteins—complex substances that make up about 90 percent of the nonwater, nonfat weight of soft tissue. Occasionally, other complex substances formed from sugars, termed *polysaccharides*, act as antigens. Haptens are relatively simple organic compounds that can combine with a protein, thus creating a new molecular species that acts as an antigen. Almost all drugs, and many substances present in foods, can act as haptens in a small percentage of people. Thus, as an example, some people become sensitive to penicillin. In them, penicillin or a substance formed from it in the body probably combines with protein present in the body to form an antigen, and, as a result, they form antibodies against this "foreign" compound. When they are exposed to penicillin again, if the same "foreign" antigen is formed, antibodies present react with this antigen and the patient then experiences a penicillin reaction. This may take any one of several forms: a shock-like state (which may cause death), skin rashes, difficulty in breathing, and so on.

In one type of hypersensitivity, the antibodies formed appear fairly soon after exposure to the antigen, and they circulate freely in the blood. This is the type of "immunity" that is produced by effective administration of a bacterial or viral vaccine, or that may occur as a result of infection. When a disease-producing organism gains entrance into an immune individual, the antigens in the organism react with the circulating antibodies, and often this process aborts the disease.

In other cases, this type of hypersensitivity (often termed the "immediate type," and characterized by the presence of effective antibodies in the plasma or serum) may cause disease. Thus the common allergies, such as hay fever, asthma, and sensitivities to foods and drugs, are examples of immediate hypersensitivity. The other type of reaction to antigens, known as "delayed hypersensitivity," is characterized by reactions between antigen and sensitized cells that occur in the tissues rather than in the blood. The reaction of sensitized cells

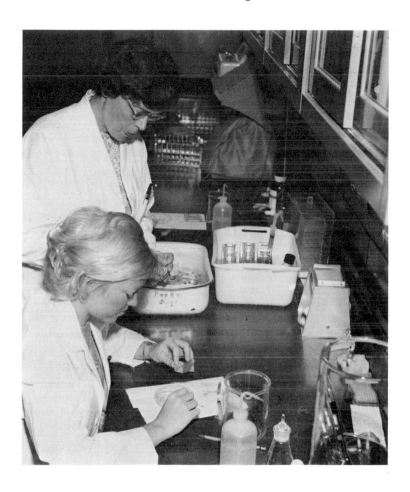

These scientists are isolating from the spleens of mice single cells, which will be used in screening tests thought to be useful in predicting the clinical effects of new compounds in allergy and other forms of hypersensitivity. (W-LRI)

with antigen takes longer to develop than the reaction of antibody with antigen in immediate hypersensitivity.

When an organ (for example, a kidney, heart, or liver) is transplanted from a human or animal donor to a human recipient, often the body of the recipient will "reject" the transplanted organ after a few weeks. This rejection is caused by a reaction between the antigens in the implanted organ and sensitized cells formed in the body of the recipient. It is necessary to suppress the ability of the recipient to form these sensitized cells, therefore, if the organ is to survive and remain functional. The physician attempts to accomplish this by giving drugs that suppress the formation of sensitized cells—generally speaking, the same drugs that are used in the chemotherapy of cancer. Thus, some of them are highly toxic, and they must be used carefully.

Another major difficulty encountered in organ transplantation is that the suppressive drugs used to prevent the formation of sensitized cells also suppress the mechanisms that produce serum antibodies. These latter are important in the resistance to infection, and often the patient may succumb to infection even though the transplanted organ still is viable (living) and functioning. It is not surprising, then, that many laboratories are searching for new drugs that can suppress the appearance of delayed hypersensitivity without suppressing the development of useful antibodies.

Another experimental method for slowing the rejection of transplanted organs by the recipient involves the use of an antiserum known as ALS (antilymphocytic serum). This antiserum contains antibodies (contained in a plasma protein fraction called globulin) that can destroy lymphocytes (white blood cells that can produce antibodies). ALS is prepared by injecting lymphocytes from human thymus, lymph node, and spleen into a horse. The horse develops antibodies capable of destroying human lymphocytes. The serum taken from the horse is fractionated, yielding a purified solution of gamma globulin that is rich in antibody. When ALS is injected into a patient before and after an organ is transplanted into his body, many of his lymphocytes are destroyed. This suppresses temporarily his mechanism for making sensitized cells active against the transplanted organ, thus giving it an opportunity to establish itself in its new environment. This therapeutic agent, like those taken by mouth, has the disadvantage that the patient's ability to form useful antibodies also is suppressed. Thus there is the danger that the patient may succumb to infection. The experience with ALS is too limited at this time to predict its eventual place, if any, in therapeutics. Autoimmune diseases, caused by delayed hypersensitivity, are diseases in which the body apparently has formed sensitized cells against antigens that are *not* foreign, but rather are naturally present in the body of the patient. This may happen, at least in some cases, because the antigen, although present in the body, does not come in contact with the cells that can be sensitized during fetal life. If contact does occur after the body "learns" to make cells sensitized against foreign antigens, cells active against the body's own tissues may be formed. As an example, the thyroid gland contains many follicles, or hollow spaces, in which a protein known as thyroglobulin is present. Apparently this protein does not leave the follicles normally and thus would be recognized by the cells active in immunity as a "foreign" protein. If, then, some of this protein does leak into the blood, cells are sensitized against it; these sensitized cells then attack and destroy tissue in the thyroid gland. This condition is classified as allergic thyroiditis.

Systemic lupus erythematosus is an example of delayed

hypersensitivity. This disease may at times resemble rheumatoid arthritis. It is a disorder that involves the smaller blood vessels and connective tissues. Lesions commonly form in the skin, the heart, lungs, kidneys, lymph nodes, and spleen. Bacterial invasion of the body sometimes causes delayed hypersensitivity. Rheumatic fever (a disease that may damage the heart) and glomerular nephritis (a disease of the kidneys) are examples of diseases that probably are caused by this mechanism.

Another important medical problem is the relative loss of function of the immediate antibody-forming mechanism in many older people. They often die of infections, such as pneumonia, that usually can be treated successfully with antibiotics in younger people. The reason seems to be that the antibiotics hold the invading organisms in check long enough for the patient's own body to make antibodies that destroy them. If this immune mechanism is not working, the antibiotics often cannot overcome the infection.

The drugs presently used in treating the diseases caused by hypersensitivity are the antihistamines and compounds (corticoids) related chemically and biologically to cortisone and cortisol (hydrocortisone). Antihistamines are designed to neutralize histamine, which is a substance released when antigens and antibodies combine with each other in the body; they are not very effective against serious allergic states such as asthma. The corticoids are more effective, but they are not curative, and when used for long periods of time may cause serious side effects.

Obviously the hypersensitivity diseases are of major importance, and many laboratories are trying to find effective drugs in this area of disease. Drugs designed to suppress delayed hypersensitivity without suppressing useful antibody formation also are on the "most wanted" list of research directors in the pharmaceutical industry.

Obesity is not a disease, of course, although obese people *are* more likely to develop heart disease and diabetes mellitus than nonobese people, and millions of Americans want to avoid or combat obesity for aesthetic reasons. The immediate cause of obesity is overeating. That is to say, if more calories of food are eaten than are used for growth or energy purposes, the excess is converted to fat and stored in the body tissues.

Why do people eat too much food and thus become obese? Only a few years ago, it seemed almost self-evident that the cause was to be found in the psychological makeup of the person and not in the physiologic and chemical reactions that took place in his tissues. Probably it is true that most obesity is brought about by such psychological factors as poor eating habits, frustrations, and overeating as a substitute when social, business, or sexual desires are not satisfied. Many Americans expend very little energy in physical exercise, and this lack of exercise is a contributing factor.

On the other hand, some scientists suspect that abnormal

Although this cat, a small electrode implanted in his feeding center, has eaten his fill (left), he immediately rushes to his food dish and eats as though starved when a weak current is applied through the electrode. (W-LRI)

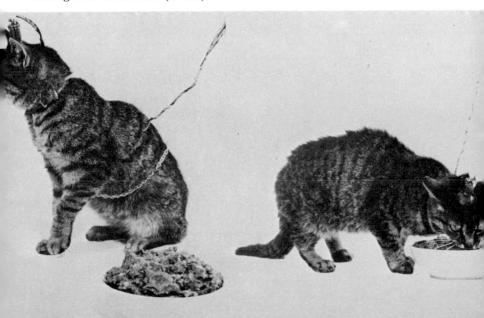

physiologic or biochemical mechanisms may play a role in some people. It is not uncommon, for example, to find that a person who is overweight by 100 pounds does not gain weight for long periods of time. In other words, he is eating only enough food to maintain, but not to increase, his body weight. It might be supposed, then, that if he managed to lose the excess 100 pounds by dieting, he could maintain himself at the lower weight just by eating the amount of food he was accustomed to when he was obese. All too often, however, some unconscious mechanism causes him to eat *more* food than this until he has regained the lost 100 pounds. Frequently, when this weight has been regained, once again his intake of food becomes only enough to maintain his weight. This type of individual seems to have some kind of regulator in his brain that almost forces him to maintain a body weight that is undesirable medically and esthetically. If a drug could be found that would "reset" this control mechanism at a lower body weight, it would indeed be a valuable therapeutic agent.

Tiny twin *feeding centers* are located in the hypothalamus (located in the subcortical portion of the brain). If an electrode is implanted in one of these in an experimental animal (usually a cat), it can be stimulated with a mild electric current. If this is done at a time when the animal is not hungry, perhaps even asleep, he immediately begins to eat. Located nearby in the hypothalamus are the twin *satiety* centers. If one of them is stimulated electrically, a hungry, feeding animal immediately ceases to eat. The satiety centers thus appear to act as physiologic brakes for the feeding centers. If the satiety centers of rats are destroyed surgically, the animals become so obese (as a result of almost constant eating) that they may become unable to stand.

For many years, drugs related to amphetamine (an ingredient of "pep pills") have been used to inhibit appetite. Most of these drugs stimulate the higher brain centers, and patients ingesting them usually exhibit psychic stimulation, restlessness, nervousness, and insomnia. Undoubtedly this mental state contributes to a relative lack of interest in activities such as eating, but some evidence indicates that they also have the effect of inhibiting the feeding center, perhaps by stimulating the satiety center.

Some years ago, scientists in the Warner-Lambert Research Institute studied a compound that inhibited the appetite of animals without causing the increased activity resulting from the ingestion of amphetamine and related compounds. Further work indicated that the probable cause of the inhibition of feeding was a stimulation of the satiety centers. This compound, chlorphentermine hydrochloride, is marketed by Warner-Chilcott Laboratories under their trademark, Pre-Sate. In humans, drowsiness and sedation are observed as frequently as nervousness and insomnia. Many patients are not conscious of any side effect. When such patients lose weight, some of them are inclined to believe that the drug had nothing to do with it because "When I take this tablet every morning, I don't feel a thing. Sure, I lost weight, but that was because I decreased the amount of food I ate." It thus may be possible to develop a drug in this area that is effective and yet not maximally satisfying to the patient psychologically.

Carbohydrates (starches and sugars) present in the diet are converted to glucose, a sugar, in the body. Glucose is the major fuel that is "burned" (oxidized) to yield the energy needed for muscular contraction. Insulin, a hormone made by special cells in the pancreas, facilitates the entrance of glucose into the muscle cells, where it is stored as muscle glycogen. This substance undergoes a complicated series of reactions that furnishes the energy for muscular contraction. Now insulin also is necessary for the formation of fat from glucose. Some scientists have postulated that some obese people preferentially use insulin to store fat, thus reducing the amount of this hormone available for muscular reactions involving glucose. In the absence of sufficient sugar, fat can be used for energy purposes. Let us suppose, as a postulate (unproved guess), that some of these people have an impaired ability to use their stored fat for energy purposes. Obviously, they would have to eat more food under these circumstances to provide enough glucose for energy purposes. Also, if the supply of insulin available for reactions involving glucose becomes too low, some glucose cannot gain entrance into the muscle cells and will be excreted in the urine. In this case, the patient will be considered to have a mild case of diabetes mellitus.

The word *diabetes* is derived from a Greek word meaning "to cross over" or "to pass through." Its modern English meaning is "any one of a number of conditions characterized by the secretion and excretion of excessive amounts of urine." *Mellitus* is derived from Latin; literally, it means "of honey." Diabetes is a disease in which there is an increased flow of urine that has a honey-sweet taste. (Older physicians actually tasted the urine of patients suspected of having the disease.) The level of glucose in the blood is high even when the patient is fasting; when this level exceeds the patient's renal (kidney) threshold, it "spills over" into the urine.

The cardinal signs of diabetes mellitus, learned early by every medical student, are the "three p's"—polyuria (increased flow of urine); polydipsia (increased intake of water); and polyphagia (increased intake of food). The glucose (responsible for the sweet taste) excreted in the urine is, of course, dissolved in water, and hence an increased amount of water is excreted along with the glucose (polyuria). This excessive loss of water causes the increased thirst (polydipsia). The loss of glucose, a valuable food, causes the patient to increase his intake of food to compensate for its loss (polyphagia). It was thought for many years that diabetes mellitus was caused by a failure of the pancreas to produce sufficient insulin. It seems evident today, however, that this is true for only about 20 percent of the known 4 million diabetics in the United States. When the disease is caused by a true pancreatic deficiency, it usually develops early in life and is known as growth-onset, or juvenile, diabetes. All of these patients require insulin for control of the disease.

Maturity-onset diabetes usually occurs after the age of 40 years, and most commonly, appears in overweight individuals and frequently can be treated without insulin. In some cases, weight reduction without drugs causes a disappearance of the signs and symptoms of the disorder; in other cases, synthetic drugs can be used. One group of drugs, the sulfonylureas, acts by stimulating the pancreas to release more insulin. Tolbutamide (Orinase, Upjohn), tolazamide (Tolinase, Upjohn), chlorpropamide (Diabinese, Pfizer), and acetohexamide (Dymelor, Lilly) are sulfonylureas. Another useful synthetic drug, phenformin hydrochloride (DBI, USV Pharmaceutical Corporation), is not a sulfonylurea and does not act by increasing the production of insulin; according to its manufacturer, "it may be considered an orally active insulin-supporting or reinforcing agent." There is some evidence that this agent interferes with insulin's role in increasing the deposition of body fat, which would increase the amount of insulin available for glucose metabolism. This explanation for the activity of the drug is supported by the finding that patients taking it tend to lose weight.

It is important that patients with diabetes mellitus be treated adequately. An acute complication, diabetic coma, can cause death if insulin is not injected promptly. Atherosclerosis often appears in patients who have been diabetics for 15 years or more; coronary disease thus is common in older diabetics. Some patients also develop diabetic neuritis, characterized at first by tingling and numbness of the hands and feet, although later, pain of a constant aching type may develop. Infections of the skin (boils, carbuncles) are common, and diabetic retinitis may result in impaired vision.

In research programs designed to explore possible causes of obesity other than simple overeating, almost inevitably the scientists directing them consider also the related problems of diabetes mellitus. I am sure that a number of laboratories, both inside and outside the pharmaceutical industry, are active in these twin fields of research.

           ◦§ ੬◦

Chronic bronchitis is a long-standing disease of the bronchi —the "tubes" that convey gases into and out of the lungs. Coughing and shortness of breath often accompany it. When infection or serious bronchial obstruction persists, bronchiectasis, atelectasis, or emphysema may develop. Bronchiectasis is characterized by dilation of the bronchi, usually with secondary infection; commonly there is abundant sputum and paroxysmal attacks of coughing. Atelectasis is a shrunken, airless state of a lung, or part of a lung, its chief cause obstruction of bronchi. The air trapped behind the obstruction is absorbed, leading to the airless state. If the absorption is rapid, there is pain on the affected side, breathing becomes difficult, and cyanosis (bluish tinge in the color of skin and mucous membranes, caused by insufficient oxygen in the blood), rapid heart beat, and shock may ensue. If the development of atelectasis is slow, increasing difficulty in breathing and weakness are the most important signs. Probably emphysema is second only to heart disease as a disabling condition. In it, there is pathologic enlargement and overdistention of the lung alveoli (air sacs at the ends of the bronchioles, the small terminal branches of the bronchi) and small bronchioles; usually its patients have a long history of smoking cigarettes, chronic coughing, wheezing, and expectoration. Difficulty in breathing often is extreme, especially on exertion; the disease is progressive and often terminates in death.

The principal drugs used in the treatment of this group of lung diseases are bronchodilators, antibiotics, and corticosteroids. A number of laboratories are searching for new bronchodilators relatively free of the side effects typical of the agents now available—nervousness, restlessness, insomnia, rapid heart beat, and, sometimes, fluctuations in blood pressure. Possible experimental models that might be useful in screening compounds for potential effectiveness in the treatment of emphysema are under investigation.

ᴄᴓ5 ᴄᴓ·

A peptic ulcer is a circumscribed erosion of the mucous membrane of the esophagus (rarely), stomach, or duodenum (first portion of the small intestine), most commonly in the duodenum. Pain is characteristic, is related to the digestive cycle, and usually occurs one to four hours after meals, and often awakens the patient at night. Attacks are most common in the spring and in the fall. Periods of exacerbation often can be related to emotional tension, excessive use of alcohol, fatigue, and dietary indiscretion. There still is disagreement about the primary cause of peptic ulceration, but no doubt that an increased secretion of acid gastric juice is an important factor in causing pain and in preventing healing. The digestive enzymes (mainly pepsin) in gastric juice, which are most active in an acid environment, may play a role also.

The drugs used in the therapy of peptic ulcer are intended

to neutralize acid, decrease the secretion of acid gastric juice, and inhibit the painful muscular spasms that may occur. Sedatives or tranquilizers may be used to reduce nervous tension and allay anxiety. Effective antacids are available, but ordinarily they do not remain in the stomach in active form for more than 40 minutes or so, and thus must be taken frequently. A long-acting antacid would be a valuable new drug.

The drugs most commonly used to inhibit secretion of gastric juice and spasm of the gastrointestinal musculature have biologic properties similar to those of atropine. The newer synthetic drugs have been developed with the objective (only partially achieved) of retaining desirable activity without the distressing side effects produced by atropine. These side effects include difficulty in starting the flow of urine, dryness of the mouth, and mydriasis (dilation of the pupils of the eyes, which may cause some blurring of vision). The first two synthetic drugs of this type were marketed in 1950—methantheline bromide (Banthine, Searle) and dicyclomine hydrochloride (Bentyl, Merrell). A number of such drugs have been marketed since, but none of them is free of the undesirable side effects. For this reason, research in this area is still quite active.

Gastrin is the name given to a substance made by the pyloric end (near where the stomach joins the small intestine) of the stomach. It causes the stomach to secrete gastric juice and to become more motile. Some laboratories are searching for synthetic compounds that will antagonize gastrin, thus reducing gastric secretion and increased gastric muscular activity.

⋙ ⋘

During the first half of this century, one of the most profitable and useful therapeutic research endeavors was the search for new vitamins. No new vitamin has been discovered for a number of years, however. Other nutritional products, such as preparations rich in protein or in unsaturated fatty acids, have been introduced in the past as therapeutic agents. At present, however, there is little interest in these agents and also little interest in nutritional research in the pharmaceutical industry.

Only a few American pharmaceutical companies have an interest in the discovery and development of drugs for the treatment of tropical diseases. I think two major reasons account for this lack of interest. Such drugs, although potentially extremely important medically in terms of world-wide need, would have little or no sale in the United States. In those companies with which I have been affiliated, the International Divisions have discouraged such research on economic grounds. They have concluded that, in the areas of greatest medical need, the patients who required these drugs could not afford to purchase them.

Some have argued that research in this area should be undertaken in spite of a lack of commercial interest. Is it right, they say, not to try to solve serious medical problems because of commercial considerations? But the research director usually sees no moral issue involved in a decision not to enter the field. After all, unless additional funds are made available (and usually they are not), introducing a new program of research in tropical diseases would necessarily decrease the research effort in those diseases that kill or cause illness in Americans. Nor is the matter so pressing as it might otherwise be, for several European countries, whose political and commercial ties to the "underdeveloped countries" are closer than those of the United States, are conducting substantial research in drugs for the tropical diseases.

◄§ §►

Most pharmaceutical research groups have been unwilling to undertake research that is financed by the government. In most cases, the work that interests the government is not product oriented; even if it is, there is little likelihood that useful products will be developed, and almost certainly the company would not have an exclusive patent position. One government-financed project, for example, involved the production (by research personnel) of relatively large quantities of old compounds that were to be evaluated in outside research organizations as potential cancer chemotherapeutic agents. Space—or, more properly, lack of it—is a problem faced by the research director: he seldom thinks he has enough. Ordinarily, the government is unwilling to pay for capital investments, such as new equipped laboratories, and therefore, accepting a government-sponsored project involves either building new facilities at company expense or reducing the space allotted to the company-sponsored program.

Often a scientist in a pharmaceutical research group can work on more than one program at a time, and allocations of his time to different projects are estimates. When the US pays the bill, however, it is preferable to hire or to segregate personnel to work exclusively on the governmental program. Otherwise there will be problems with the auditors and accountants assigned by the government to follow the financial aspects of the program. Often frequent and voluminous reports on the progress of the research program are requested by the governmental sponsor: somebody has to prepare these reports, and all too often only the scientists themselves are in a position to do so. This not only is a job they do not relish, but it also decreases the time that they can spend on experimentation. If the government-sponsored program is terminated, another problem arises. The research people who have been working on the project then must be absorbed into the company program at company expense—or terminated. If the problem involves a sizeable number of scientists, abrupt termination can cause serious morale problems in the company research organization.

◄§ §►

Of course, this rather brief survey of potential research programs is far from complete. Some therapeutic agents not discussed are respiratory stimulants, anesthetics, anthelmintics (drugs used to kill or eliminate intestinal worms), antiarthritics, anticoagulants (used to inhibit blood clotting), anticonvulsants (used in epilepsy), antinauseants, antipruritics (drugs used to relieve itching), enzymes, hematinics (drugs used in the therapy of anemias), hormones (except the hormone-like drugs used in contraception and insulin), and sedatives. I shall discuss in a later chapter some of my thoughts about entirely new fields of research that may lead to entirely new drugs in the future. The examples discussed in this chapter will, I hope, give some insight into the factors the research director must evaluate in establishing the research program for a pharmaceutical research group.

CHAPTER 11

Drugs Without Profit

Where Need is Great

WYETH LABORATORIES made available to the medical profession in 1968 an important new drug—important, that is, to the mere handful of patients who will benefit from it. From a commercial point of view its only importance, if any exists, lies in the "public relations." The drug is an antivenin (antiserum) to combat the toxin of the North American eastern coral snake, found only in nine southeastern states. Wyeth has sent supplies to poison control centers located in Texas, South Carolina, North Carolina, Mississippi, Louisiana, Arkansas, Alabama, Florida, and Georgia. In addition, a central supply has been deposited with the National Communicable Disease Center in Atlanta. The antivenin is available without charge to physicians who request it.

For many years, the ethical pharmaceutical industry has supplied drugs that are useful, often life-saving, in the treatment of diseases too rare to create a commercially profitable market. Always there has been an obvious, although small, need. The company meeting this need often has had a research program or line of products that made it fairly easy to provide the drug. When I went to Sharp & Dohme in 1942, the company owned hundreds of horses, used to prepare antisera against various diseases, particularly tetanus (lockjaw), a disease of high fatality and great military importance. The tetanus organism abounds in soil and animal feces; wounds, including powder burns, offer ingress into the body. During the early years of World War II, the only effective way to protect patients against this threat was to inject potent antiserum. Today almost every child—and certainly every military recruit—is immunized with tetanus toxoid (vaccine). When preventive therapy is indicated, a "booster" dose of toxoid is given. The patient's body responds by pouring into the blood antibodies against the tetanus organism, and thus antiserum (containing such antibodies) is not required.

But to return to our story. A few people who required tetanus antiserum were highly sensitive to horse serum. For them, the injection of antiserum made from the horse was a dangerous procedure, and to meet this medical problem, Sharp & Dohme made tetanus antiserum using cattle rather than horses, and supplied this product for the small number of patients who required it. It was removed from the market a few years ago because tetanus antiserum made from the blood of immunized human volunteers became available commercially.

The availability of horses and trained personnel also prompted Sharp & Dohme to develop a series of antivenins (antisera) against snake venoms and black widow spider venom. The snake antivenins were transferred to Wyeth Laboratories some years ago and now are supplied only by that organization; however, Merck Sharp & Dohme Laboratories still supply the black widow spider antivenin. Although production of this product was discontinued in 1945 with an inventory sufficient to last until 1952, the obvious need of the few patients involved caused the company to resume production in 1954. These antivenins are marketed despite the fact that only 2,000 to 3,000 cases of snake bite poisoning occur each year in this country, and the known incidence of black widow spider bites is between 1,500 and 2,000 cases annually.

In some cases, companies have deliberately undertaken research and development projects to supply a drug useful only in treating a rare disorder, even though the new product did not fit directly into the skills existing in the organization. In part, at least, this was true in the development of products designed to be used in the management of the disorder known as phenylketonuria. The story of phenylketonuria began to unfold in Norway in the early 1930s. A mother of two mentally retarded children noticed, as others did, that these children had a peculiar odor, since described in other cases as musty, horsy, or barn-like. A number of physicians examined the children but were unable to explain the odor. Finally the mother enlisted the help of a biochemist, Dr. Asbjørn Følling, a distant relative. He found that a green color was produced when ferric chloride was added to the urine of these children, and also succeeded in isolating a compound known as phenylpyruvic acid from their urine. Using the ferric chloride test, he discovered eight additional cases within a few months, and described his findings in the medical literature in 1934. The name, phenylketonuria, was coined later when it was known that several abnormal chemicals in addition to phenylpyruvic acid appear in the urine of patients with the disorder. Some of these compounds belong to a series known to chemists as phenylketones.

It is estimated that about one in every 20,000 live infants is born with the disease. In the United States, the incidence is approximately 200 new cases annually. It occurs equally in both sexes, is rare in people of Negro or Jewish ancestry, and blue eyes and blond hair predominate.

In the first months, these children appear normal in behavior. But at about four months of age they begin to show signs of mental retardation, and the disease is full blown by the age of two or three years. Clinically they have low grade intelligence, awkward gait, tremors, epileptic seizures, and frequently, a skin disease, eczema.

Proteins consist of a number of smaller substances, known as amino acids, chemically combined with each other. One of these amino acids, phenylalanine, exists in the blood of phenylketonurics in concentrations that are 15 to 20 times the usual level. Normally, phenylalanine is converted to another amino acid, tyrosine, in the body. But patients with phenylketonuria are born without the enzyme required for this chemical reaction; as a result, phenylalanine builds up in the blood and is transformed into various other substances that are excreted in the urine. The green color produced with ferric chloride is due to the presence of phenylpyruvic acid; the odor, really in the urine, and which develops only after the urine has stood for an hour or so, is due to phenylacetic acid, produced from one or more of the abnormal substances in the urine.

Further investigations indicated the probability that most of these infants would develop normally if they were given a diet low in phenylalanine. The proteins in normal foods contain too much of this amino acid to make it practical to select ordinary foods for this purpose, but special diets were developed by two pharmaceutical companies. Ketonil, the trademark used by MS&D for its preparation, was a powder that was mixed at home with oil or shortening, sugar, and water to make a liquid or paste. The other product was marketed later by Mead Johnson & Company. Trademarked Lofenalac, it was packaged in such a way that one standard measure added to two fluid ounces of water made a nutritionally complete preparation equivalent to 20 calories per fluid ounce. The Mead Johnson preparation turned out to be more acceptable to the patients and their parents. Consequently, Merck Sharp & Dohme deleted Ketonil several years ago from its manufacture.

Certain organic chemical molecules have the property of binding metals and are termed *ligands*. The complex formed when a ligand binds a metal is known as a *chelate*, derived from the Greek term, *chele*, which means the claw of a lobster. Just as the pincers, or claw, of the lobster grasps its prey, so do the chemical groups of a ligand molecule grasp a metal to form a chelate. One of the chemical warfare agents available, but never used, during World War II was lewisite, an oily organic liquid substance containing carbon, hydrogen, chlorine, and the metal, arsenic. Even tiny amounts on the skin were irritating and slightly larger amounts caused death. An English chemist, Sir Rudolph Peters, and his associates developed a compound that would form a chelate with the arsenic and thus neutralize the lewisite. This substance commonly is referred to as British antilewisite, or BAL. Although BAL was not used in chemical warfare, it has proved useful in the treatment of poisoning by the heavy metals, arsenic, gold, and mercury. When it is injected intramuscularly, it forms chelates with the metals and transports them from the body. This drug in peanut oil solution, now known as dimercaprol injection, is marketed by Hynson, Westcott & Dunning under the name, BAL in Oil.

◦§ §◦

Only a few thousand cases of acute metal poisoning are diagnosed and treated in the United States annually, and lead poisoning is responsible for most of these. However, some authorities estimate that 125,000 to 225,000 children are poisoned each year. Most of these victims are children living in slum areas who have chewed and swallowed old flaky paint, which usually contains white lead. In 1935 the German chemist, F. Munz, patented a ligand with the jaw-splitting name, ethylenediaminetetraacetic acid, understandably commonly shortened to EDTA. He used it to form chelates with calcium, which, by keeping the calcium in solution, was useful in the technology of fibers and textiles. It did, however, form chelates with a number of metals.

The first published case of acute lead poisoning treated with a derivative of EDTA occurred in Children's Hospital in Washington, DC, in June, 1951. The patient was a 3-year-old boy, who had absorbed enough lead to have convulsions and to show signs of damage to his brain. Dr. Samuel P. Bessmond and Dr. Hugh Ried, who had the biochemical advice of Dr. Martin Rubin of Georgetown University, decided to try out EDTA as a therapeutic agent. The derivative used contained sodium (to neutralize acidity and to solubilize) and calcium (to avoid depletion of calcium from the body). A series of doses was given at frequent intervals, and the patient clinically was well on the third day.

A solution of the sodium calcium derivative of EDTA now is known as calcium disodium edetate injection. It is marketed by Riker Laboratories under its trademark, Calcium Disodium Versenate, and can increase the excretion of lead in the urine by a factor of 40. If an amount of lead as small as 3 milligrams (about one ten-thousandth of an ounce) were circulating in the blood, death might result. With EDTA, this amount can be lost in the urine in a short time. Tablets of the calcium disodium edetate also are available, and are used as follow-up therapy after the course of injections, and sometimes given to patients who have no clinical evidence of lead poisoning but who present laboratory evidence that their bodies contain excessive amounts of lead.

◄§ §►

Scleroderma is a rare disease of unknown cause that starts with a painless watery swelling of the skin. Over a period of months or years, the skin hardens, shrinks, and becomes immobile, and then appears smooth and shiny, the face assuming a mask-like appearance. The tight skin may lead to difficulty in using the extremities. Often calcium salts are deposited in the skin. Spontaneous recovery has been observed, especially in children. But usually the disease slowly progresses, often with periods of remission. In some cases, improvement in terms of skin softening and mobility have been brought about by injecting the disodium salt of EDTA intravenously daily for a few days. Presumably, the beneficial effect is due to the chelation of calcium and its removal from the skin. Treatment is tricky, because removal of too much calcium from the body can cause dangerous toxicity. The drug used for this purpose, known as disodium edetate injection, is supplied by Abbott Laboratories, whose trademark is Endrate. Three thousand patients received this drug in 1967.

జ్ఞ ఆ

Probably about 2,000 cases of poisoning by iron occur in the United States each year. When the poisoning is severe, the death rate may approach 50 percent. One author estimates that in the US at least a dozen people die annually of iron intoxication, most of them children who have eaten sugar-coated tablets of iron salts used in the treatment of anemia. Deferoxamine mesylate (Desferal mesylate, CIBA) was approved for marketing by the CIBA Pharmaceutical Company in April, 1968. It is a specific iron-chelating agent, and (as a drug) is used only for the therapy of iron intoxication. It is administered by intramuscular injection. According to CIBA, only three of 467 patients who received the experimental drug died.

జ్ఞ ఆ

Wilson's disease is a rare inherited disorder, from which about 1,000 persons in the United States are known to suffer. In this disease, abnormal amounts of copper are deposited in several organs, which results in degeneration in the brain, liver, and kidneys. Tremors, uncoordinated movements, and evidences of liver damage are present, and children with the disease die within a few years. Copper is transported in the plasma as a constituent of a blue protein known as ceruloplasmin. In Wilson's disease, the level of ceruloplasmin in the plasma is extremely low. Probably this lack of transporting protein accounts for the accumulation of copper in the tissues.

Penicillamine first was obtained from a broth containing degraded penicillin. For a time it was hoped that it might be used as an intermediate for the synthesis of penicillin, but this proved to be impractical. In 1956, Dr. J. M. Walshe, now at Cambridge University in England, obtained some penicillamine from MS&D. He reported that it could be used orally in the therapy of Wilson's disease. Other chelating agents (BAL and EDTA) had been used for this purpose, but they were not active by mouth. MS&D marketed penicillamine under their trademark, Cuprimine, in August, 1963. Treatment of patients with this drug usually causes at least some improvement in liver function: tremors are less marked and frequent, and movements become more controlled. Some patients return to their jobs and other routine activities.

In 1963, British investigators found that penicillamine also is useful in the management of patients with another rare inherited disease, known as *cystinuria*. Patients with this disease excrete in the urine abnormally large quantities of the amino acids, cystine, lysine, arginine, and ornithine. The loss of these substances from the body does not cause any known harmful effects: three of the four amino acids are soluble and cause no difficulty in the urinary tract. However, cystine is not very soluble and precipitates to form kidney and bladder stones, the only known pathology in cystinurina. Penicillamine is useful in the treatment of this condition, not because it is a chelating agent, but because it reacts chemically with cystine in the body to form two soluble substances, which prevent the formation of the cystine kidney and bladder stones.

✍ ❧

Cancer is a term that includes a large number of malignant (life threatening) diseases. In most cases it occurs as a tumor (solid clump of tissue), but in some cases, such as the leukemias, the cancer cells float freely in the blood and body fluids, and even invade tissues. Cancers often metastasize—that is, cancer cells of the original tumor migrate to other regions of the body where they locate and multiply. As a rule, cancer cells multiply more frequently than normal cells, and uncontrollably. Some of the drugs that have utility in combating cancer really inhibit cell multiplication. The trick is to give enough drug to inhibit the division of the cancer cells without inhibiting necessary cell multiplication in normal tissues. Obviously, overdosage with such a drug will cause toxicity. The differences between different kinds of cancer are illustrated, of course, by the different clinical and anatomical characteristics of each type. It is not surprising, perhaps, that some drugs appear to have activity against only one, or at least a limited number, of cancers.

✍ ❧

Multiple myeloma is a rare type of cancer. Probably about 5,000 cases exist at any given time in the United States. In this malignant disease, bone and bone marrow are invaded by a type of cancer cell termed the myeloma cell. The bones of the chest and the skull are involved most frequently, abnormal proteins often appear in the urine, and pain is the outstanding complaint and may be the only symptom—usually localized in the chest, and aggravated by motion or deep breathing. As the ailment progresses, typical signs of a wasting, malignant disease appear. Patients with the disease usually first notice pain when they are in their late fifties. The disease is rare before the age of 35 years, and is almost twice as common in men as in women.

Melphalan, marketed by Burroughs Wellcome & Company under their trademark, Alkeran, is useful in the treatment of multiple myeloma. Approximately one third of the patients show a favorable response, although none is cured. The drug is not recommended for the treatment of other types of cancer.

∽§ ?∾

On February 10, 1968, the mother of 4-year-old Marek Maziarz, in the town of Nowa-Sól, Poland, observed a growth in the boy's lumbar region, and he was taken to a hospital in Zillona-Gora, where it was found he had a kidney tumor (cancer). The tumor was removed surgically, and the region was irradiated, but it was felt that treatment with a drug marketed by MS&D also should be used.

Back in Nowa-Sól, "ham" radio operators Julius Schmidt and Andrezej Grigo radioed an international appeal for the drug. Their signal was picked up by Fernand Dubret in Cheserex-by-Nyon, Switzerland, on February 24. Dubret enlisted the help of a Geneva journalist, Raoul Riesen. That same night they contacted pharmacist Albrecht Rochat, at the Canton Hospital in Geneva. He sent 3 ampuls of the MS&D drug on the 9 PM flight to Paris to connect with a flight to Warsaw the next morning. Marek's father, Alfred Maziarz received the package at 11:30 PM on February 25.

The cancer growing in the body of little Marek Maziarz was a Wilms' tumor, which accounts for about 20 percent of all cancers found in children. It first develops in the kidney, but often metastasizes (spreads) to the lungs and liver. Often it is discovered by the mother when she is bathing the child; in later stages, weight loss, anemia, weakness, and gastrointestinal disorders appear.

Actinomycin D is an antibiotic that was discovered by Dr. Selman A. Waksman at Rutgers University. As a drug, it is known by its generic name, dactinomycin, and was marketed as Cosmegen by MS&D in 1965. Its primary use is in the treatment of Wilms' tumor, although a few other rare tumors of muscle, testes, and uterus show some temporary response. MS&D estimates that fewer than 10,000 persons in the United States have tumors that will respond to the drug. Dactinomycin was the drug that went so swiftly from Switzerland to Poland.

Ten years ago, about two thirds of the patients with Wilms' tumor died in spite of surgery and irradiation. Today the combined treatment with surgery, irradiation, and dactinomycin has resulted in the survival of as many as 80 percent of patients in some hospitals.

✍️ 🍃

On July 27, 1966, Abbott Laboratories released to the market a new drug useful only for the treatment of two rare diseases involving the blood. The drug, trademarked Vercyte, is known generically as pipobroman; it is used in polycythemia vera and chronic granulocytic leukemia. Abbott estimates that about 1,000 patients are receiving the drug at any one time.

Polycythemia vera is a disease characterized by a great increase in the number of red blood cells circulating in the blood; usually there is also an increase in cell volume in the bone marrow (where red blood cells are manufactured) and in the size of the spleen. The cause is not known. Ordinarily it occurs during middle or late life, is most common in males, and Jews are especially susceptible. About 5,000 new cases of the disease occur in the United States annually. Patients with polycythemia vera tend to bleed easily and to form blood clots in their blood vessels, and occlusion of the coronary vessels of the heart or of the cerebral (brain) blood vessels may cause death. Survival times of 10 to 15 years after diagnosis are not uncommon, however.

Chronic granulocytic leukemia is a form of cancer that occurs most commonly between the ages of 20 to 40 years, and is characterized by an increase in the number of granulocytes (a type of white blood cell) in the blood. Excessive production of these granulocytes occurs in the bone marrow, spleen, and liver, and they may infiltrate other tissues, such as the mouth, intestine, kidneys, lungs, joints, lymph nodes, and the spinal cord and brain. Weakness, fatigue, pallor, loss of appetite, and weight loss are noticed by the patient, and often a low-grade fever. The disease progresses and always is fatal; the average survival time is three to four years, although 2 percent of patients live longer than ten years. There are approximately 3,500 new cases of the disease annually in the US. Remissions tend to occur oftener and to last longer when the patient receives the Abbott drug.

Another drug used in the therapy of chronic granulocytic leukemia is hydroxyurea, marketed by Squibb Beech-Nut as Hydrea. It is used also in the management of patients with melanoma. Malignant melanoma is an uncommon form of cancer; it accounts for about 1 percent of deaths from cancer.

The original tumor originates in the pigment-forming cells of the skin, usually at the site of a mole, and almost all cases occur in white people. The cancer grows with great rapidity and metastasizes to many organs, especially the liver, lungs, heart, and brain. Most of the lesions are pigmented, but some are not, and the disease is fatal in two to four years. Rare cases have been cured when the cancer has been discovered before metastases have formed.

ᥫ᠍ᠣ ᠍ᡝᥫ

Fungi are plants, many of them microscopic, that do not manufacture chlorophyll, the green pigment of the higher plants, nor can they manufacture their own food. They obtain the materials necessary for energy and growth by breaking down dead plant and animal tissues or by infecting living organisms, including man, thus often causing disease. Molds, mildews, yeasts, rusts, smuts, mushrooms, and puffballs are examples.

Athlete's foot and ringworm are common fungal infections of the skin and nails. *Candida albicans*, a yeast, causes infections in the mouth (thrush), nails, skin, vagina (vaginal moniliases), and anus. This type of infection, limited to the external surfaces of the body, though troublesome, usually does not threaten life. Rarely, fungi invade the body and cause systemic infection. These infections develop slowly, but usually produce death after months or years. Invasion of the body by *Histoplasma capsulatum* does not always cause clinical disease, and many thousands of persons infected by it have only symptomless calcifications in their lungs.

The antibiotic, amphotericin B, marketed by Squibb Beech-Nut, Inc., as Fungizone Intravenous, and the only therapeutic agent available for the treatment of systemic fungal infections, has made possible the successful treatment of previously hopeless fungal infections. This drug is extremely toxic, and must be used with strict medical supervision of the patient. Often injections must be given daily, or on alternate days, for several months. Squibb Beech-Nut supplied about 78,000 vials of the drug in 1967. Since a single course of treatment requires a large number of vials, only a small number of patients were involved. Amphotericin B is not effective against diseases caused by bacteria.

~§ §~

During operations on the heart, in which blood is bypassed through special machines in order to obtain a bloodless operative field, acidosis often develops—a condition in which the blood is too acidic. Acidosis is present also in cardiac arrest, that is, sudden stoppage of the heart beat, sometimes a causative factor in arrest. Acidosis can kill by preventing the transfer of oxygen from the blood to the cells or by stopping the heart beat.

In December, 1965, Abbott Laboratories marketed a drug that is useful—even life saving—in combating the acidosis accompanying or following cardiac bypass surgery and cardiac arrest—known as tromethamine with electrolytes; the Abbott trademark is Tham-E. This drug neutralizes the excess acid in the blood. It also causes an increase in the flow of urine, which results in the loss of some electrolytes, particularly sodium chloride and potassium chloride, from the body. (Electrolytes are compounds that conduct an electric current when they are dissolved in water.) For this reason, the dosage form used contains tromethamine (to neutralize acid) and the electrolytes, sodium chloride and potassium chloride. The trademark is derived from the complex chemical name, Tris (Hydroxymethyl)-Amino Methane; the E on the end stands for electrolytes.

Other drugs, such as sodium bicarbonate and sodium lactate, have been used to combat acidosis. Tromethamine, however, has advantages. It is less upsetting to other chemical balances within the body and has the ability to enter cells, so that it can exert its antacid effect within the cells themselves.

Tromethamine was made first by chemists of the Commercial Solvents Company, and was used commercially as an emulsifying agent in waxes, cosmetics, and polishes. In the late 1950s, Dr. Gabriel G. Mahas, then at the Walter Reed Institute for Medical Research, began experimenting with a purified form of the compound, and interested Abbott in undertaking its development in 1959. It was studied clinically for six years by over 400 investigators prior to marketing. Sometimes stored blood in blood banks becomes too acidic; Tham-E neutralizes the excess acid.

◅§ §▻

Patients with the rare liver disease, primary biliary cirrhosis, itch continually, day and night. So agonizing is this itching that some are driven to thoughts of suicide; most of the patients are women in their thirties or forties. Despite the serious nature of the disease, most victims do not feel very ill and may live ten years or more with the disease—if they can stand the terrible itching. Normally the liver pours bile into the intestinal tract; the bile acids present in this fluid help in the digestion and absorption of fats. Much of the bile acid entering the intestine is reabsorbed through the intestinal walls and goes back to the liver, while some stays in the intestine and is eliminated.

In primary biliary cirrhosis there is a partial blockage of the flow of bile from the liver to the intestine. Under these circumstances, extra amounts of bile acid seep into the blood and eventually reach the skin in relatively high concentrations. When this happens, the almost unbearable itching occurs. Cholestyramine, a whitish powdered resin, taken orally, brings marked and continuous relief from itching in most patients with primary biliary cirrhosis. MS&D's trademark for this drug is Cuemid. This substance is not absorbed from the intestinal tract; it combines with bile acid in the intestine and carries it away from the body in the stool. This prevents the reabsorption of bile acids, thus preventing a marked increase in the level of these substances in the blood and in the skin. Cholestyramine was marketed in 1965.

◄§ §►

Herpes simplex keratitis (dendritic keratitis) is a disease of the cornea of the eye, caused by a virus. Ninety percent of untreated cases progress to the stage of large, deep ulcers that interfere with vision. It is an uncommon disorder; Dr. Dan M. Gordon, a New York ophthalmologist, estimates that a small fraction of 1 percent of all eye patients have the disease. The affected cornea has a branched lesion resembling the veins of a leaf, with knoblike terminals. The early signs include foreign-body sensation, excessive secretion of tears, sensitivity to light, and reddening of the white of the eye. Before drug therapy became available, the only treatment was the removal of the infected cells by cautery or surgery.

Some years ago, scientists at Yale University were investigating a substance now known as idoxuridine that interfered with cell division; they were interested in its possible utility in preventing the growth of experimental cancers. In 1961, Dr. Herbert E. Kaufman, Chief of the Division of Ophthalmology of

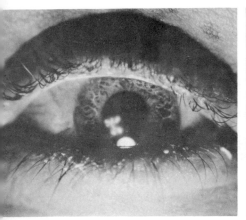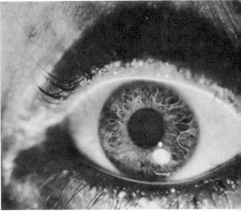

Symptoms of herpes simplex keratitis, a viral disease that can result in visual impairment, were present for four days when examination revealed a dendritic ulcer on the corneal epithelium. (Left, before.) Treatment with Stoxil (idoxuridine, SK&F) was initiated. (After.) On the seventh day of treatment, the dendritic ulcer had completely healed; treatment was terminated after ten days. Idoxuridine was the first effective therapeutic agent for a true viral disease. (SK&F)

the University of Florida College of Medicine, began to study this compound's possible effectiveness in preventing the multiplication of the virus responsible for herpes simplex keratitis. In 1962, he and his associates reported to the New England Ophthalmologic Society in Boston that idoxuridine "resulted in a prompt cure of dendritic keratitis in rabbits and was completely nontoxic." The next step, of course, was to test the drug in patients with the eye disease. It worked. In Dr. Kaufman's words:

> The results were simply dramatic. No one who has ever seen patients with these acute eye conditions, knowing what the progressive course of the disease can be, can imagine our reaction when we literally saw the disease disappearing.

Another problem remained: the new drug was unstable and soon decomposed. Dr. Kaufman enlisted the support of a pharmaceutical company, which was able to devise stable dosage forms suitable for topical application. As a matter of fact, three pharmaceutical companies began studies of the drug in the laboratory and in the clinic. It was marketed in 1963 by Smith Kline & French Laboratories (Stoxil); Alcon Laboratories, Inc. (Dendrid); Allergan Pharmaceuticals (Herplex). The discovery that idoxuridine is effective against this disorder was a milestone in the history of medicine. This drug is the only therapeutic agent marketed for the *treatment* of an infection caused by a true virus. Applied topically to the diseased eye, the drug will abort the disease in almost all cases.

Addison's disease is a progressive ailment caused by underactivity of the cortex (outer portion) of the adrenal glands. It is characterized by increasing weakness, weight loss, low blood pressure, dehydration, gastrointestinal upsets, and an abnormal increase in the color of the skin and mucous membranes, and sometimes, by a low level of blood sugar. The disease is rare; about one person in 250,000 in the United States has it. The adrenal cortex secretes two types of hormone. One, typified by aldosterone, has a marked effect on the excretion of electrolytes; even small doses produce a marked retention of sodium by the body and an increased excretion of potassium salts in the urine. Two, typified by cortisol, does not have such a marked effect on sodium and potassium salts, but does have the property of increasing the deposition of glycogen (a storage form of sugar, "animal starch") in the liver.

Fludrocortisone acetate is a synthetic compound that has the biologic properties of aldosterone. It is marketed by Squibb

Beech-Nut, whose trademark is Florinef Acetate. This drug, together with cortisol (or another drug having the biologic properties of cortisol) is used only in the treatment of patients with Addison's disease.

◄§ ξ►

Some drugs of limited commercial potential are marketed either because some physicians wish to use them or because they are used in those situations in which other standard agents fail. The disease involved may or may not be rare. Two drugs of this class are arginine glutamate (Modumate, Abbott) and monosodium L-glutamate (Glutavene, Crookes-Barnes). These drugs are designed specifically for the treatment of hepatic coma.

Bacteria in the intestinal tract break down proteins to form ammonia and other toxic nitrogen-containing substances. When these substances are absorbed into the blood, they are transported to the liver, where they are converted into harmless compounds. When the liver is severely damaged, these detoxification reactions do not occur, and the ammonia and other toxic substances pass into the general circulation; when they reach the brain in sufficient concentrations, the sympton complex known as hepatic coma results. Patients with hepatic coma have flapping tremors of the hands and are confused or actually unconscious. Attacks are brought on in patients with liver disease if large amounts of protein are eaten, or if bleeding occurs in the intestinal tract. Treatment involves restricting proteins in the diet, correcting bleeding if it is present, and administering antibiotics to inhibit intestinal bacteria. Ammonia is detoxified in the body by its conversion to urea, a harmless waste product that is excreted in the urine. Glutamic acid and arginine are key compounds required for the formation of urea in the body. Injection of the two drugs, Modu-mate and Glutavene, is designed to remove ammonia from the blood by hastening its conversion to urea.

◈

Barbiturate poisoning is familiar to everyone, although the incidence is not so high as many people suppose. According to one estimate, 12,000 cases occurred in 1964. In addition to the procedures normally used in treating this condition, some physicians believe that administration of drugs that stimulate the higher nervous centers are useful. Several drugs will do this; two of them are marketed more or less specifically for use in barbiturate poisoning: bemegride (Megimide, Abbott), marketed in 1958, and ethamivan (Emivan, USV Pharmaceutical), marketed in 1961. Abbott's product was used in the treatment of about 4,000 patients in 1967.

◈

Shock is a serious clinical situation requiring immediate treatment. It has diverse causes: major surgery, injury, massive bleeding, coronary attacks, overwhelming infection, poisoning, and some drug reactions, and is characterized by a state of circulatory collapse with a marked fall in blood pressure. Insufficient blood returns to the heart from the tissues, and thus there is a deficient flow of blood from the heart to the tissues.

Several drugs used in treating shock have been available for a number of years. The newest entry is an interesting substance known as angiotensin amide. It was marketed as Hypertensin by CIBA Pharmaceutical Company in June 1962. Under certain circumstances, the kidneys secrete into the bloodstream a protein known as renin, which reacts with a protein in the plasma to form angiotensin I, a decapeptide—that is, a compound formed by the chemical union of ten amino acid molecules. Angiotensin I then is converted to angiotensin II, an octapeptide (formed by the chemical union of eight amino acids), by another plasma protein. Angiotensin II is the most potent hypertensive (bloodpressure raising) substance known: doses as small as one microgram (about one thirty-millionth of an ounce) given intravenously per minute in man will cause a marked rise in blood pressure.

Angiotensin amide differs only slightly in chemical structure from the natural angiotensin II. The biologic properties of the two compounds are identical. Angiotensin amide is recommended for cases in which the blood pressure must be restored with a minimum of delay, and during procedures, such as surgery, when support of blood pressure becomes necessary. It has not been evaluated in shock caused by coronary thrombosis.

◆⧉ ⧉◆

Some drugs are used for the diagnosis of disease states rather than as therapeutic agents. A good example of such a drug, used in the diagnosis of a rare clinical disorder, is metyrapone, marketed by CIBA Pharmaceutical Company, whose trademark is Metopirone, in January, 1962. The pituitary gland is a small structure connected to the base of the brain. Its anterior (front) lobe manufactures several hormones that travel at intervals in the blood to various other endocrine (hormonal) glands, which are stimulated to secrete the hormones they manufacture into the bloodstream. Sometimes the pituitary gland loses its ability, at least partially, to produce its hormones, thus causing a state of partial hypopituitarism or limited pituitary reserve. One of the hormones secreted by the pituitary gland is ACTH (AdrenoCorticoTropic Hormone). This substance stimulates the cortex (outer portion) of the adrenal glands (one is perched atop each kidney) to manufacture, among other compounds, cortisol (hydrocortisone), an important hormone. As the level of cortisol rises in the blood, the secretion of ACTH is inhibited. When the blood level of cortisol is low, the secretion of ACTH is stimulated. This is a good example of an automatic biologic feedback mechanism.

ACTH really causes the formation of precursors of cortisol, and the drug, metyrapone, blocks the final synthesis of cortisol from these precursors. When it is given to normal people, it causes a large continuous secretion of ACTH because the level of cortisol in the blood naturally is very low. The precursors of cortisol are excreted in the urine and can be determined chemically. If the pituitary gland is normal and is secreting ACTH, the level of these substances increases when metyrapone is given to the patient. If, on the other hand, the patient's gland is underactive (partial hypopituitarism) the administration of the drug does not cause an increase in the urinary level of cortisol precursors.

◄§ §►

No one knows precisely how many "drugs without profit" are supplied by the pharmaceutical industry. If all drugs sold without profit are included, the number is very large indeed. However, those drugs that are specific for the treatment of rare diseases are the ones that are of real importance. Some pessimists predicted that the marketing of these medically valuable drugs would cease following the passage of the Kefauver-Harris Amendments in 1962. Time has proved them wrong, because several important drugs of this type have become available since then. I am sure the pharmaceutical industry will continue to generate them in the future.

Coda

A THIRD OF A CENTURY AGO there were no tranquilizers, no sulfa drugs, no antibiotics, no contraceptive drugs, no corticoids, few vitamins, no antihypertensives, no antihistamines, no orally effective diabetic drugs, no prophylactic drugs for gout, no potent orally active diuretics, no drugs to lower the level of cholesterol in the plasma, no vaccines against poliomyelitis, measles, or mumps. Today we have all of these drugs and more. Most of them have been discovered and developed by the pharmaceutical industry. Some people, observing this imposing list of therapeutic agents, have wondered whether research in this area has not reached a point where there are not too many more potent drugs to be discovered in the future. This is truly a naive point of view. The drugs now available represent a very small fraction of the therapeutic agents needed for the effective treatment and prevention of diseases. With rare exceptions, drugs now available are curative in only two areas of disease: some (far from all, unfortunately) infectious diseases, and diseases caused by vitamin deficiency (rare in this country). We do not have curative drugs for, indeed do not even know the fundamental causes of, the major killers, coronary disease and cancer. With one minor exception (a drug effective against herpes simplex keratitis), we have no agents effective against viral diseases, probably the leading cause of illness and of absenteeism from work. True, we have drugs effective in lowering blood pressure, but we cannot cure it and do not know its cause. Drugs that are useful in crippling and troublesome illnesses such as arthritis, mental disease, and allergy are only palliative, not curative. Drugs that are effective in the management of patients with diabetes mellitus, and for the prophylaxis of acute attacks of gout, are available, but we cannot cure either disease.

Obviously, then, the drugs that will be discovered and developed in the future far outnumber those made available in the past. It is impossible to predict what drugs will appear in the next quarter of a century. The truth of this statement becomes evident if we imagine that we are living in 1945 and are predicting the drugs that will be available in the next quarter of a century. Of course, some of the modern drugs were predicted 25 years ago, but this was because everybody was an optimist in those early days. Some sulfa drugs were on the market and penicillin was undergoing development. Most executives in research management, including myself, simply recited the major medical problems and predicted that effective drugs in these areas of disease would appear within 25 years. Thus, we anticipated a cure for cancer, for viral diseases, for atherosclerosis, for schizophrenia, and so on. How wrong we were.

I am more conservative today. I think it will be a long time before really effective, curative drugs will be found for noninfectious, nonnutritional diseases. Even in the area of infection, the cure of viral diseases will, I think, elude us for many years to come. It will continue true in the future, as in the past, that many drugs will be found unexpectedly, either in the laboratory or in the clinic. But we cannot escape the fact that discovery really hinges on the biologic evaluations that are used in searching for new drugs. If we use the same ones in the future that we use today, the chances of finding entirely new types of drug will be minimal. We *must* somehow develop new, different, clinically meaningful procedures.

New methods of evaluation of potential drugs can be devised only when basic research has advanced to a state where scientists interested in the development of drugs can use them in establishing new procedures. A good example of what I mean is illustrated by the discovery of chlorothiazide (Diuril, Merck Sharp & Dohme), the first of an important series of agents useful in removing excess water and sodium salts from the body and in combating high blood pressure. During the 1930s, university scientists worked out in considerable detail the mechanisms employed by the kidney in forming urine, the major medium for the elimination of waste products from the body. In the late 1930s and early 1940s, methods of measuring the different activities of the kidney were devised. All of this was basic information, and had no obvious connection with product development.

In 1944, the Sharp & Dohme scientists, Dr. Karl Beyer, a biologist, and Dr. James Sprague, a chemist, decided to use this basic information about the kidney to search for the drug now known as chlorothiazide. The biologists on Dr. Beyer's team used trained dogs as test animals. The various parameters of kidney function were measured in these animals before and after administration of new compounds synthesized by Dr. Sprague and his associates. Research can be agonizingly slow and unpredictable, and chlorothiazide did not reach the market until 1958, fourteen years after the search for it started in the laboratory. The important point, however, is not that it took so long to find and market the new drug, but that it was possible to find it at all only because of the background of basic research available.

We must recognize several facts about basic research. First, most of it must be conducted in universities, research insti-

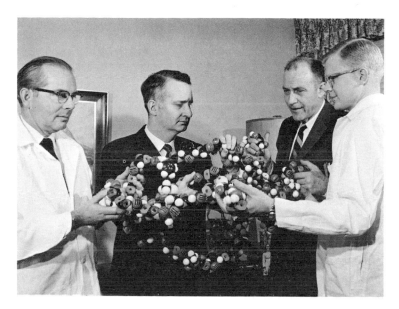

Senior members of the 20 Merck chemists who synthesized in the laboratory bovine pancreatic ribonuclease hold a model representing a single molecule—Drs. Frederick Holly, Ralph Hirschmann, Robert Denkewalter, and Daniel Veber. This is an example of basic research. Ribonuclease and the chemical substances made during its synthesis have no known use as drugs, but almost surely the knowledge gained will lead to new therapeutic agents. (MS&D)

tutes, and governmental research facilities such as the National Institutes of Health. Probably in the future, as in the past, much of the money for basic research must come from the government. The resources of the pharmaceutical industry are far too small to cope with the huge problems that can be solved only with more basic information. Second, we—including pharmaceutical top management—must recognize that all research inherently is inefficient. All working scientists know this. They are inclined, therefore, to do those things about which they feel most certain. In the area of basic science, this leads to many small advances, or even to horizontal maneuvers that do not truly represent advances. Breakthroughs occur only when scientists have, in a sense, taken a research gamble that paid off, or when a scientist has a flash of intuition that enables him to fuse a number of bits of information into a coherent whole. Third, how much basic information is needed before it can be used intelligently in the discovery of a drug? The answer is simply that it must reach a level where the discovery of the new drug is *feasible*, not *certain*. In view of the basic information available, however, the direction that the scientist should go becomes clear.

As an example, the discovery of chlorothiazide was feasible in view of the basic information available. It was not certain, in 1944, that a useful drug could be found, but, to repeat, certainly it was feasible. The search for a drug to cure schizophrenia, on the other hand, is not feasible at present. We do not have enough fundamental information about this disease, and if a curative drug is found in the near future, it will be a lucky accident. Fortunately, lucky accidents in the field of drug research have occurred in the past and probably will occur again in the future.

Dr. Albin M. Weinberg, Director of the Oak Ridge National Laboratory, has compared science and basketball:

> I like to draw an analogy between science and basketball. Our high school basketball coach used to say, "In setting up a good shot at the basket, by all means keep the ball moving. It doesn't matter so much where the ball moves as long as it does not remain in one place; only in this way are openings created." This approach to basketball is certainly inefficient; the amount of wasted motion is much greater than the amount of motion specifically directed at the goal. And yet by following this prescription our team won most of its games. In the same sense science is inefficient; by maintaining scientific ac-

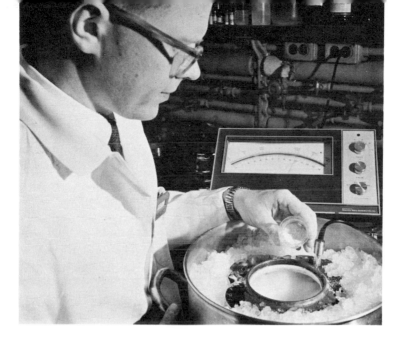

A chemist helps synthesize the enzyme ribonuclease, announced simultaneously by the Merck Sharp & Dohme Research Laboratories and Rockefeller University. High-speed mixing speeds delicate reactions and gives higher yields of peptides. (MS&D)

tivity in areas that are broadly of interest, one creates opportunities that can be exploited practically. . . .

A number of areas of basic research are important for the future discovery of drugs, though admittedly, many of them have not yet reached the stage of feasibility. Some of these have been discussed in Chapter 10.

≈§ §≈

In the higher animals, including man, a new life begins when a spermatozoan fertilizes an ovum (egg) by uniting with it. It is a fact—almost an incredible fact—that this single cell contains all the coded information necessary to produce a living, functioning animal. This information comes from both parents, and can, in turn, be transmitted to the offspring of the new animal. Every living cell, then possesses a "code of life," often called the genetic code, that enables the cell to produce the enzymes required for the chemical syntheses and reactions necessary for life. Proteins exist as large molecules made by the chemical union of a number of smaller molecules known as amino acids. There are about 20 different amino acids, but many protein molecules consist of several hundred amino acid residues arranged in a definite sequence. This long chain of amino acids is coiled in a way characteristic for each protein, with a definite three-dimensional structure and a definite kind of surface. Now some, although not all, of the proteins in the body are enzymes. Enzymes are the expert "chemists" that bring about essential chemical reactions in the tissues with an ease that mocks the skills of human chemists. The architecture of their surfaces is such that they can combine with smaller chemical molecules and bring two or more of them into contact with each other so that a chemical reaction occurs. The new substances thus formed are released, and the same enzyme molecule is available to repeat the process many times.

The coded information required to make enzymes and other proteins resides in huge linear molecules present in the nuclei of cells. These macromolecular substances are known collectively as DNA (DeoxyriboseNucleic Acid). The long chain is made up of alternating chemically united molecules of phosphoric acid and deoxyribose (a sugar); an organic (carbon-containing) base is connected chemically to each sugar residue. (The term residue is used to mean chemically combined molecule.) Two of these bases belong to the class of organic compounds known as purines, adenine and guanine. Two others are the pyrimidines, cytosine and thymine. If all the DNA in one human cell could be spliced together to form a single thread, it would be about 36 inches long and weigh about 6 picograms. (One billion picograms is equivalent to approximately one thirty-thousandth of an ounce.) The chromosomes that can be observed during cell division are strands of DNA, and each human cell normally contains 46 of them. Genes are regions in the chromosome that contain the coded information required for the synthesis of a single specific protein.

In cells that are not dividing, the DNA usually is present as two long chains or loops coiled around each other like the strands in a piece of rope. This coiled structure is referred to as the DNA helix. The spatial relationships are such that the adenine in one chain is paired with the thymine in the other, as cytosine and guanine are also paired. During cell division, the two chains uncoil, much as a zipper does when it is unfastened. As this goes on, each chain acts as a template, or mold, along which a new DNA chain forms. Thus, when division is completed, the number of DNA chains has doubled, so that each daughter cell contains a DNA helix identical with that of the parent cell.

Although the genetic code resides in the DNA, which is in the nucleus of the cell, the actual synthesis of enzymes and other proteins takes place outside the nucleus in the cytoplasm (extranuclear part of the cell). DNA in the resting (non-dividing) cell acts as a template for the synthesis of another type of macromolecule known as RNA (RiboNucleic Acid). The sugar in RNA is ribose, and the organic bases are the purines, adenine and guanine, and the pyrimidines, cystosine and uracil. As the RNA chain is formed along the DNA template, adenine in the DNA chain pairs with uracil in the forming RNA; thymine in DNA pairs with adenine in RNA; and cytosine in DNA pairs with guanine in RNA. As the RNA is formed, it peels off and separates from the DNA template.

The code for a single amino acid is determined by a sequence of three bases in the RNA molecule. Thus, the sequence of three uracil residues is the code for the amino acid, phenylalanine. If the RNA formed as just described is the messenger that will transmit the information required for the synthesis of a protein containing 200 amino acid residues, obviously it must be long enough to possess 600 bases. Thus, messenger RNA molecules are very large on a molecular scale. Messenger RNA migrates into the cytoplasm where other RNA molecules, known as transfer RNA, are present. Transfer RNA molecules contain about 70 bases. These molecules are bent to form a helix, but at one end have three unpaired bases. These unpaired bases are the code for one of the 20 amino acids involved in protein synthesis. Each transfer RNA molecule carries with it a single amino acid residue.

When protein is synthesized, the bases of the transfer RNA become loosely attached to the bases in the messenger RNA. Adenine, remember, pairs with uracil, guanine with cytosine. Thus, if a region of messenger RNA has three uracil bases, a transfer RNA molecule whose unpaired bases are all adenine will combine with this region. In this way, the amino acids are lined up in proper sequence to form a specific protein molecule.

The actual union of these amino acid residues to form the protein takes place on the surface of structures known as ribosomes. A ribosome moves along a strand of messenger RNA just as a pulley can be pulled along a horizontally stretched piece of rope. As each triplet code reaches the ribosome, it combines with the appropriate triplet in a transfer RNA molecule. This is repeated when the next triplet reaches the ribosome, and the two amino acid residues thus brought together combine with each other. Thus the string of combined amino acids becomes longer and longer as the ribosome moves along the messenger RNA chain. Eventually the complete protein is formed, each amino acid having been incorporated in proper sequence.

It is obvious that changes in the DNA—for example, the presence of the wrong base at a particular site—will result in the production of abnormal proteins. If a portion of the DNA strand is lost, it may be impossible for the cell to manufacture an essential enzyme. These molecular changes can lead to disease or even to death. Diseases caused by defective formation, or lack of production, of enzymes are known as diseases of enzymic defect or as inborn errors of metabolism. Some of them—Wilson's disease, phenylketonuria, cystinuria— were discussed briefly in Chapter 11. A large number of such diseases are recognized, and the list grows longer each year.

Hemoglobin is the red protein in the red blood cells that carries oxygen from the lungs to the tissues. Slight imperfections in the DNA in some people cause the formation of slightly different hemoglobin molecules; more than 65 slightly different hemoglobins have been found in humans. The hemoglobin present in patients with sickle-cell anemia has a valine residue instead of the glutamic acid residue normally present at one site in the huge molecule. In this disease, the normal disc shape of the red blood cells changes to a crescent (sickle) shape when the oxygenated hemoglobin in them loses oxygen as a result of exposure to lowered oxygen pressure. Approximately 8 percent of the Negro population in the United States has red blood cells that can be made to sickle in the laboratory. Sickling occurs in the body when the oxygenated hemoglobin loses its oxygen to the tissues; the nonoxygenated hemoglogin actually crystallizes in the red blood cells and distorts them. The rate of red blood cell destruction in the body is rapid, and this causes anemia (too few red blood cells and too little hemoglobin). Few patients with clinical evidence of this disease live beyond 40 years.

If somehow we could learn to modify the code contained

in DNA, the possibilities for improving the human race are enormous, though admittedly, some modifications might prove to be disastrous. But, if we knew enough, conceivably we might modify the DNA in a spermatozoan and an ovum prior to fertilization. This might take the form of correcting a defect in one parent and thus preventing a disease in the offspring. Or, it might be that the DNA could be improved so that the offspring was a person of much higher intelligence than either parent. Perhaps it could be so arranged that some of the genes coincided with those of the world's finest musicians, artists, or scientists. This is dreaming, but some day, perhaps a century from now, the dream may become reality. This possibility horrifies some, delights others.

We know now that morphological changes in the DNA in the intact animal, including the human, can be caused by some drugs and by overexposure to x-rays. We do not yet know whether these changes will be reflected in abnormalities (or the contrary) in the offspring of those persons whose DNA has been so changed. Will it ever be possible to devise drugs that will modify the DNA in living people in desirable ways? I think the answer is *Yes*, but I also think that this will not happen for a long, long time. In the meanwhile, it is very important that basic research in this area continue, so that the information necessary for the development of this type of drug can be accumulated.

❦

Another important area of basic research has to do with the problem of aging. Why do we grow old? Why do some microorganisms live for minutes or hours, some animals for years, other animals for decades, some trees for centuries? Nobody knows. We have all read about cells in tissue culture that live on year after year. But do they? Actually no single cell that has not divided to produce new progeny lives more than a limited time. In a way, the new cells that result from cell division are analagous to babies in a human population: they live for a time characteristic of the cell or until they divide to form new cells. Meanwhile, "old" nondividing cells die, just as old humans do.

From the biochemist's point of view, the known changes that take place as people or animals become older are meager. The amount of water in the body and in the tissues decreases with advancing age. This, perhaps, is obvious even without chemical analysis: the wrinkled, leathery skin of older citizens attests to it. Tissues, especially subcutaneous tissues, contain many fibers composed of a protein known as collagen. As animals age, these fibers tend to unite with each other by the formation of cross linkages. This uniting tends to limit mobility and function.

Actually, humans must be concerned with three different kinds of aging. We age biologically, psychologically, and socially. Biologic age refers to our position on the path from birth to old age and death. Psychologic age refers to our capacity to learn, remember, and respond effectively to our environment. Social age refers to our habit systems or social roles. Most studies in aging have been concerned only with the study of the biologic type. It is evident, however, that it would not be useful to find means of increasing the life span of humans if the resulting old people could not think or remember adequately and could not take care of themselves or interact socially with other people. Brain cells do not divide and renew themselves. And so the brain may suffer more than other tissues from the ravages of time.

At a scientific meeting held in New York in May, 1968, Dr. Holgar Hyden of the Institute of Neurology, University of

Goteborg, Sweden, suggested a possible way to rejuvenate aged brain cells. The DNA in brain cells does renew itself at intervals, and many opportunities for mistakes during its continuous synthesis may occur as the animal grows older. Thus, the DNA synthesized later in life may contain mistakes that cause impaired memory, learning, and social behavior. Dr. Hyden and his associates prepared DNA from the brain of one animal and injected it into the brain of another. The injected DNA apparently functioned since the rate of synthesis of protein in the recipient increased by 100 percent in one hour. Biochemical analysis showed that the injected DNA was incorporated in the brain cells of the second animal. Presumably the increased rate of synthesis of protein was caused by this new DNA. As Dr. Hyden stated, "this does not mean that an elixir of life has been found."

A number of things we do not know. For example, what kind of protein was formed? Is it functionally valuable· or is it "nonsense" protein? How long will the injected DNA remain active? Will it duplicate itself in the new environment? Dr. Hyden is an optimist. He believes that some day it will be possible to replace old, mistake-ridden DNA with fresh, ordered DNA. Perhaps this can be done by wrapping up the new DNA in a harmless virus that will take the DNA into the brain cells. Studies of aging have not reached a point where it is feasible to discover new drugs in this area. This is one field of basic research that has been relatively neglected.

❦

For many years, science fiction writers, and others as well, have been interested in drugs, as yet undiscovered in real life, that can affect the mind in desirable ways. Will we discover drugs that will improve memory, decrease the learning period, increase concentration? Research in this field is quite active, although I think that finding a new drug at the present time would have to be classified as a lucky event. In 1966, Dr. N. Plotnekoff, a scientist working at Abbott Laboratories, published the results of his studies with magnesium pemoline. This compound, first synthesized in Germany, was known as a mild stimulant of the central nervous system. Dr. Plotnekoff placed rats in a box whose floor was a grid that would conduct an electric current. After 15 seconds, a buzzer sounded for 15 seconds. During the last 5 seconds of the noisy period, a mild electric shock was given by electrifying the grid. The animals could escape the shock by jumping to a platform outside the box.

When untreated rats were treated in this fashion, after seven trials they learned to escape from the box before they were shocked. Rats treated orally with magnesium pemoline learned to escape after only two or three trials. Twenty-four hours later, the treated animals still escaped in three to eight seconds. At this time, untreated controls required a much longer time to escape, although on the average they too escaped before the shock. Two other drugs known to stimulate the nervous system (types of "pep pills"), methamphetamine and methylphenidate, did not affect the rate of learning and the duration of memory in these rats. I have been told that magnesium pemoline was given to humans with no measurable beneficial effect. The animal experiments do offer hope, however, that an effective drug may be found in the future.

In 1965, evidence that a learned response could be transferred from one rat to an untrained one by injecting RNA from the trained rat into the peritoneal cavity (body cavity housing the gastrointestinal tract) of the untrained one was published. Rats were trained to approach a food cup when a click was presented. RNA extracted from their brains was injected into untrained rats, who then showed a significant tendency to approach the food cup when they heard the click. Some scientists have failed to confirm this report, but others seem to have done so; at present, the evidence is inconclusive. In the end, if it turns out that learning can be transferred in this way, it probably means that the learning process causes formation of a "memory protein." RNA, as I indicated earlier, acts as a template for the formation of protein, but, intuitively, this solution seems too simple.

Puromycin is an antibiotic that interferes with the production of protein by bacteria and by animals. Dr. B. W. Agranoff and his co-workers at the University of Michigan studied the effect of this substance on memory formation in goldfish. A rectangular tank containing water was divided into two equal halves by a barrier that reached to within an inch of the surface of the water. The goldfish were placed in the tank on one side of this barrier. That side then was illuminated for 20 seconds, after which an electric shock was given through the water. The fish could escape the shock by swimming over the barrier to the other side of the tank. A positive response (that is, evidence of memory formation) was recorded when the fish swam over the barrier in time to escape the shock. After 21 to 30 training periods, 50 percent of positive responses occurred.

Now puromycin was injected into the fluid surrounding the brain. This obliterated improvement after the first trial. Puromycin thus blocked memory formation, presumably by preventing the synthesis of a "memory protein." If the antibiotic was given one or two hours after trial 20, no memory block occurred, presumably because the "memory protein" already had been synthesized by that time. After numerous experiments, Dr. Agranoff concluded that fish receiving puromycin were alert and were able to solve short problems: they could recall past events, but could not form permanent memory for new events.

Russian scientists have used a different experimental approach. They trained rats to escape an electric shock by moving in a maze when a bell was sounded. When an enzyme (ribonuclease or RNAase) that causes the destruction of RNA was injected into the brains of trained rats, the rats no longer escaped the shock when the bell was sounded: in other words, there was a loss of memory. DNAase, an enzyme that causes the destruction of DNA, did not cause the loss of memory. However, if it were injected prior to the training period, the rats did not learn to escape the shock. This was expected, because DNA is the template for the formation of RNA; in its absence, RNA and hence new protein could not be formed. As expected, also, the injection of RNAase just prior to the training period prevented establishment of a positive response, presumably because a "memory protein" could not be formed in the absence of RNA.

At a meeting of the American Psychiatric Association in Boston in 1968, Dr. Samuel Bogoch presented evidence that learning and memory may be correlated with the synthesis of new glycoproteins (proteins to which a sugar is combined chemically) in the brain. Two of these glycoproteins were found at the beginning of a learning process, and the third appeared in the memory phase. Carrier pigeons were used as experimental animals. Dr. Bogoch said that he and his co-workers also had data indicating that the levels of glycoproteins in cerebrospinal fluid (which bathes the spinal cord and brain) increased when psychotic patients improved and decreased when the disease recurred or became worse.

LSD and marihuana are powerful drugs that affect the mind, though unfortunately, the changes in mental activity that they produce are undesirable and harmful. However, there is the possibility that chemical modification of these substances might produce substances with desirable effects on mentation. Several pharmaceutical groups are making such modifications of pure active compounds isolated from marihuana. I am sure that some of these will be, or are now being, studied in humans.

◄§ ε►

Schizophrenia is the most important major mental disorder. Patients with this disease account for 15 to 20 percent of first admissions to public mental hospitals and for 60 percent of the permanent hospital population. Schizophrenia begins most frequently in adolescence or early adult life, and is characterized by a progressive withdrawal from the environment, regression to a childlike or infantile type of feeling and acting, and inadequate and inappropriate emotional responses. The term "schizophrenia" means "splitting of the mind." The schizophrenic cannot meet the demands of adult adjustment and has an inadequate personality.

During the last 15 years or so, many papers describing biochemical abnormalities peculiar to schizophrenia have appeared in the scientific literature. Thus, scientists have reported finding abnormal chemicals in the blood and urine of these patients, but others have been unable often to confirm these findings. The injection of blood from schizophrenics into animals, usually rats, has resulted in bizarre or abnormal behavior. Unfortunately, this has been true sometimes when the donor of the blood did not have schizophrenia. Again nothing suggestive of a way to search for an effective drug has emerged from such experiments.

Back in 1956, Dr. Robert G. Heath, chairman of the department of psychiatry at Tulane University, and his associates reported that they had isolated a protein from the plasma of schizophrenics that did not occur in normal people. They named it taraxein. When they injected taraxein into normal volunteers, they produced a syndrome closely resembling schizophrenia. Unfortunately, as the years passed, other investigators have not been able to duplicate these results. Recently Dr. Heath and his co-worker, Dr. Iris M. Krupp, who still claim to prepare taraxein, have suggested that this protein "might be an antibody to the brain, and schizophrenia might be an autoimmune disease." In other words, they are suggesting that the schizophrenic has, for some unknown reason, made antibodies to a protein normally present in the brain. When this antibody (taraxein) reacts with the protein in the brain, the tissue is altered and schizophrenia results. They reported also, as Dr. Heath's group has done before, that monkeys receiving taraxein show behavior resembling that of humans with the disease.

It seems highly unlikely that schizophrenia is an inherited disease, although some sort of predisposition may be inherited. Dr. William Pollin and Dr. James R. Stabenau of the National Institute of Mental Health have studied a group of identical twins in which one twin is normal and the other has schizophrenia. Since both twins evolved from a single ovum, the genetic code in each should be identical. Inherited diseases are due to some defect in the genetic code—that is, to some alteration in DNA. If, indeed, the disease is acquired and not inherited, this makes it more probable that a drug effective against it may be found some day.

It should be pointed out that some psychiatrists do not accept the theory that the disease is due to some aberration in body chemistry. Indeed, Dr. Ronald D. Laing, of the Tavistock Institute of Human Relations in London, does not even use drugs in treating the disease. According to his analysis,

Schizophrenia is not a disease at all, and is not in one person, but is between people. It represents a broken down relationship, and the way to mend it is to involve the schizophrenic in a relationship that means something to him.

A number of drugs have been claimed to be useful in the management of patients with schizophrenia. For example, such diverse substances as the breakdown products of epinephrine (adrenaline), a hormone made in the body by the medulla (inner core) of the adrenal glands, and nicotinic acid, a vitamin that is curative for the nutritional deficiency disease, pellagra, have been used. Most physicians that treat patients with schizophrenia agree that the only really helpful drug, however, is one of the so-called major tranquilizers. The first of these was chlorpromazine hydrochloride (Thorazine, SK&F), the introduction of which in 1954 revolutionized the treatment of schizophrenia. This drug and a number of related ones have permitted many schizophrenics to leave mental institutions and even to resume gainful employment. There has remained a hard core of patients, however, who have not responded to any therapy, drug or psychiatric.

The new drug, thiothixene, marketed by the Roerig Division of Pfizer under the trademark, Navane, in 1967, is helping to pull these resistant patients back on the road to reality. Dr. Karl T. Dussik, of Tufts University, first investigated the usefulness of this drug in this type of patient. In a double-blind study of 45 patients, he found that the drug was most effective in the treatment of long-term withdrawn patients. Dr. Dussik then treated 103 chronic schizophrenics who had not responded in the past to any medication, 23 of whom had been hospitalized for more than 20 years. Twenty one of them, three of whom had been in the hospital for more than 30 years, improved so much that they were discharged from the hospital. Almost half of the patients responded to the drug; 15 responded "extremely well"; 16 improved markedly; and 19 responded to a lesser degree.

◦§ §◦

Scattered throughout the body are cells known collectively as the reticuloendothelial system, RES, most of which are in the liver, spleen, bone marrow, and lymph nodes. Some of them are fixed permanently in one tissue, but most are free to wander around in the body. These cells have the ability to engulf (swallow up) and destroy or remove foreign particles that gain entrance into the body. Under normal circumstances, most of these foreign particles are bacteria. However, particles of metals, plastic, carbon, and so on are engulfed by the RES cells if they are injected into the bloodstream.

A common method of measuring the degree of activity of the RES is to inject India ink, which contains supended particles of carbon, intravenously into animals, such as rats, and to measure the time required for removal of the carbon particles from the blood. The more active the RES, the shorter will be the time required. When certain bacteria—sometimes living, sometimes killed—are injected into animals, the RES is stimulated. Extracts prepared from these bacteria have been active in some cases. When the experiments have been done under carefully controlled conditions, it has been possible to show that animals whose RES has been stimulated can resist otherwise fatal exposure to some bacterial and viral infections, and that the growth of cancers implanted into stimulated animals is prevented or inhibited.

Obviously, drugs that could be used to stimulate the RES in humans might well be valuable. They have not yet been found. Many scientists are investigating the RES, however, and

I am confident that an active drug will be discovered eventually. But I am not optimistic that this will happen soon.

◄§ §►

Scientists working in the laboratories of the American Medical Association's Institute for Biomedical Research have found that an unknown substance in some foods increases the resistance of mice to typhoid. This unknown substance has been named pacifarin. Pacifarin is not an antibiotic or a vitamin; it does not kill the typhoid organism. Somehow it makes it possible for the organism and the animal host to get along together without the appearance of disease. So far pacifarin has been effective only against typhoid; however, it is possible that other pacifarins will be found effective against other diseases.

◄§ §►

Traditionally, the dentist has not written a large number of prescriptions, although of course he uses a number of modern drugs in his practice. In many cases, however, he recommends to his patients products that can be purchased over the counter without a prescription. This may explain, perhaps, the fact that most of the research in the dental area done by, or financed by, the pharmaceutical industry is sponsored by companies or divisions of companies that market proprietary (over the counter) drugs and consumer products. These investigations are most active in two areas of disease and in one area that is a social problem for many people. The diseases are dental caries (tooth decay) and periodontal disease (pyorrhea). The social problem is unpleasant breath odor.

Shortly after the teeth are cleaned by brushing, deposition of a material known as plaque begins on the surfaces of the teeth. It is formed by the growth of bacteria that produce filamentous strands. It causes the "furry" feel to the tongue that is familiar to everybody. The immediate cause of dental caries is the local production of acid by bacteria. The micro-organisms responsible for this grow well in plaque, and it is important to remove them by brushing the teeth frequently. It seems evident that one method of controlling dental caries would be to use agents that kill bacteria. At the present time, topically applied antibiotics and antiseptic chemicals are under study in dental clinics. One problem is that special methods of keeping them in contact with the teeth surfaces for appreciable periods of time must be used. If this method does reduce the incidence of dental caries, the next problem will be to devise dosage forms or methods of application acceptable to the consumer.

Recently the Quinton Company (the division of Merck & Company that markets proprietary drugs) has been cooperating with the National Institute of Dental Research in studying an enzyme known as dextranase. This enzyme catalyzes the breakdown of complex substances known as dextrans, which are high molecular-weight compounds formed by the chemical union of many glucose molecules. (Glucose exists in combined form in ordinary cane sugar, also known as sucrose.) They are made in the mouth from sugar by the bacteria (certain strains of streptococci) that also produce acid from the sugar. The dextran acts as a sort of glue to hold the plaque and bacteria on the surface of the teeth. Experiments at the National Institute of Dental Research indicated that incorporation of dextran into the diet of laboratory animals prevented dental caries, presumably by destroying the dextrans on the teeth. The acid-forming bacteria then could not adhere to the teeth and so did not cause caries. The next step is to determine whether dextranase is useful in preventing caries in humans. Opinion grows that the plaque and the bacteria growing in it are different in older people from the plaque and bacteria found in childhood and early adult life. Caries are much more common in the younger age groups. On the other hand, periodontal disease, which is the major cause of the loss of teeth, occurs much more commonly in older age groups.

Back in the 1920s, Dr. J. F. McClendon, then at the University of Minnesota Medical School, suggested that the content of fluoride in the enamel of the teeth might be correlated with resistance to the development of caries. He developed this hypothesis because he knew that the hardness of apatites, minerals resembling tooth enamel in chemical composition, was related to their fluoride content—the more fluoride present, the harder the apatite. In the early 1930s, one of his graduate students, Dr. Wallace D. Armstrong, now head of the Department of Biochemistry in the Medical School of the University of Minnesota, compared the fluoride content of the enamel of noncarious teeth with that of the remaining enamel of teeth with caries. Dr. McClendon's hypothesis was confirmed: the enamel of the healthy teeth had a higher concentration of fluoride than the enamel of the carious teeth. Other scientists studied the incidence of caries in various regions of the United States. It was found that the incidence was lowest in communities whose drinking water contained relatively high concentrations of fluoride.

Today, many communities add fluoride to their water supply. When fluoridated water is drunk regularly, especially during the period when the teeth are developing, the reduction in the incidence of caries can amount to as much as 60 percent. The amount of fluoride added is enough to give a final concentration of 0.7 to 1.2 parts per million. Fluoride solutions also are painted on the tooth surfaces by the dentist. Capsules containing fluoride and vitamins are available, and are recommended by many dentists. Some toothpastes also include compounds containing fluorine in combined form.

A number of other chemicals are being studied as agents to harden enamel and decrease its resistance to erosion by acid. These include salts of metals (calcium, zirconium, molybdenum, tin, gold) and various phosphate salts. In some cases, the metal salt has included fluoride; for example, zirconium fluoride has been studied.

Of course, diet is important. Children need adequate amounts of vitamins and minerals to form healthy, normal teeth. An excessive intake of sugar (sucrose) makes it possible for bacteria to make the dextran "glue" that binds them to the tooth surfaces, and this sugar also is converted to acid by certain bacteria. The acid erodes the enamel, causing dental caries.

Periodontal disease is a term that includes several diseases of the tissues surrounding the teeth. In serious cases, pockets of pus form around the roots of the teeth; in milder cases, it exists as a simple gingivitis, or inflammation of the gums. The disease often is accompanied by an atrophy, or wasting away, of the bony sockets, so that the teeth become loose and may fall out. There have been many theories advanced to explain the cause of periodontal disease. Regardless of the fundamental cause, most dentists agree that the regular removal of plaque and calculus (tartar) is the most effective means of preventing it. Calculus is a hard material formed by the deposition of calcium apatite in the filamentous plaque, and it should be removed by the dentist or dental hygienist at regular intervals. It is possible that dextranase may prove useful in preventing the formation of plaque and calculus in humans. If so, it should be useful in preventing both periodontal disease and caries.

Unpleasant mouth odors often are the result of eating pungent foods such as onion and garlic, which results in the presence of unpleasant odors in the expired air. In other cases, the bad odor originates in the mouth from decaying food particles, but also from bacteria and infection. Modern technics, especially a procedure known as gas chromatography, has made it possible to isolate and identify some of the substances responsible for these bad odors. It now has become feasible to search for agents that will neutralize and destroy them chemically. The "anti-odor" preparations now marketed are surprisingly effective, but those of the future should be even more efficient and long-lasting.

◆§ ॐ◆

There are some superficially related natural phenomena that I believe intuitively could help us develop exceptionally interesting drugs—if it were not for the fact that our basic knowledge about them is almost vanishingly small. To my knowledge, at present no pharmaceutical laboratory is studying them. Probably the question most often asked of physicians about sleep is, "How can I manage to get more of it more regularly?" But there are much more interesting questions. What is sleep? Why is it? What causes it? There has been much speculation about these questions, but we do not know the answer to many of them. Must something happen inside us to make us sleep? Or, conversely, must something happen to make us awaken? Or, of course, both? What is the basic natural state, sleep or wakefulness? *

The experimental use of the electroencephalograph in recent years has made it possible to investigate sleep objectively in humans. This instrument records electrical waves (brain waves, EEG patterns) of variable voltage. Trained investigators

* Perhaps the most thorough and scholarly book on sleep is that edited by Anthony Kales, MD: SLEEP: Physiology & Pathology, Philadelphia, J. B. Lippincott Company, 1969.

interpret recordings of these waves and can distinguish several patterns peculiar to sleep and to its depth. In animals, even more information can be gained because electrodes can be implanted deep into the brain. When the sleeper is dreaming, his eyes undergo rapid, jerky, rolling motions. These are known as REMs (rapid eye movements) and can be recorded as EOGs (electrooculograms, or continuous tracings of eye movements). Some EEGs (brain wave patterns) exhibit configurations characteristic of dreaming.

Now, we probably dream, on the average, about 20 percent of the time during sleep. Assuming that eight hours is the *average* duration of sleep in 24 hours, a person 60 years of age has spent 20 years asleep, four years dreaming. Is dreaming normal sleep plus the dream? Or is the dream state something different from dreamless sleep? Do the two states, dream state and dreamless sleep, have the same or different functions? We just don't know. When a night's sleep is missed, is a "sleep debt" incurred? Yes, but only in part. Most people accustomed to eight hours of sleep daily find that sleeping ten or twelve hours after missing one or two nights sleep is sufficient.

The dream state is a different matter. Volunteers have been prevented from dreaming by awaking them at every onset of dreaming. When this is done, there is a powerful stimulus to make up the lost dream time. In a typical case, a subject has six or seven episodes of dreaming during a night. If he is deprived of these episodes, probably during the second night it will be necessary to awaken him ten or 12 times to prevent dreaming. By the fifth night of deprivation, 30 awakenings may be required. Suppose a drug that would increase the duration of dreaming—or, conversely, decrease or prevent it— were found. Would it be useful? Most likely we shall not know until such an agent becomes available, as I believe it will. Objective measurements of the brain waves and REMs of animals indicate that they dream, and so a biologic test system for a drug affecting the dream state already exists.

The behavior of bears, badgers, and racoons offers an example of a peculiar sleep pattern. In the wild state, they undergo prolonged periods of sleep in the winter. During these times, their body temperatures may decrease by as much as 15°F. The heart rate decreases markedly—from the 90s to the 20s per minute, in the bear. In one published study, a sleeping grizzly bear produced a total of only 180 milliliters (less than half a pint) of urine over a period of more than three months. The three animals just mentioned are warm blooded. That is, even during the winter sleep they must maintain their body temperature within fairly narrow limits. When it tends to become too low, they "burn" stored food to maintain it. During their winter sleep, they resemble a human whose body temperature has been lowered artificially to perhaps 85°F. Some other animals undergo true *hibernation*. That is, under the stress of cold, they somehow switch from the normal warm blooded state to a cold blooded state. In other words, they simply do not maintain a relatively fixed body temperature, but, rather, their body temperatures follow variations in the environmental temperature. However, it is true that they do begin to generate body heat if their internal temperatures approach levels that threaten life.

Woodchucks, ground squirrels, hedgehogs, and hamsters are animals that undergo true hibernation. The heart rate of a hamster may decrease from 500 to 600 beats per minute to only six beats per minute during hibernation. True hibernation thus obviously differs from normal sleep. It is not surprising, perhaps, that we find little or no detectable spontaneous electric activity of the brain during deep hibernation.

A drug that would safely produce a state resembling the winter sleep of the bear, or, better, a state of true hibernation in the human, might be extremely useful. It would be especially valuable if this state could be produced without the necessity of cooling. Even if external cooling were necessary, however, a state of true hibernation would permit humans to survive at very low body temperatures for prolonged periods of time. During this time, the requirement of tissues for oxygen and food would be reduced almost to zero. This would be an ideal state for patients undergoing prolonged and difficult surgery. In this age of space exploration, controlled hibernation might increase many times the duration of space flights.

Of course we have numerous drugs that cause states resembling sleep. Their actions, in usual dosages, range all the way from mild sedation to deep anesthesia. Drugs like morphine produce stupor; barbiturates and pharmacologically related drugs, given in hypnotic doses, cause a state closely resembling sleep; lower doses of the barbiturates cause calmness (sedation) without sleep; anesthetics cause anesthesia. But it is doubtful that any of these generate entirely normal sleep. A drug that would do so would be most welcome.

We have drugs, ranging from caffeins to "pep pills," that combat sleep. Until we know more about the phenomenon of sleep, we shall not know just how these drugs work. I think we can be reasonably certain that they do not inhibit sleep by evoking the mechanisms normally used by the body for this purpose.

Hypnosis is a state that many people associate with sleep. Obviously the two states are not the same, however. The hypnotized subject ordinarily maintains his posture, and responds to suggestions made by the hypnotist. Moreover, the EEG pattern of a subject does not change as he becomes hypnotized. If, however, the hypnotist induces true sleep by means of suggestion during hypnosis, the brain wave patterns change to those typical of sleep. The important thing about hypnosis is that the hypnotized subject is in a state of heightened suggestibility. Even without hypnosis, suggestion is a potent factor in the therapy of many illnesses. If we had a drug that could heighten susceptibility to suggestion in a useful way, it might become a valuable therapeutic agent. Of course, such a drug also might be dangerous if wrongly used, but this is true of most potent drugs. It is true of life.

ও৪ ৪ু

Every now and then somebody asks me whether I believe that stocks of ethical drug companies will continue to be growth stocks in the future as they certainly have been in the past. Since I have no special knowledge of the stock market and its vagaries, I can only answer this question from the point of view of a pharmaceutical research director. I believe that the drug companies have fared well in the market place because they have provided uniquely useful products that have contributed tremendously to the health and well being of the citizens of this country—and, for that matter, of the world. I personally am optimistic that the drugs of the future will be numerous and even more valuable than those already available. I know, of course, that the drug industry is under attack by people who would like to have patents covering drugs abolished and the prices of drugs lowered. The FDA regulations and practices that have come into being since the passage of the Kefauver-Harris Amendments in 1962 have made the development of new drugs much more expensive and much slower. In spite of all this, I think the drugs yet unborn will turn out to be so useful that the pharmaceutical industry will continue to thrive and grow.

In 1941, just a few months before I went to Sharp & Dohme from the University of Minnesota Medical School, the value of a share of Sharp & Dohme stock on the New York Stock Exchange was $3.25. Suppose an investor had purchased 100 shares for $325.00. How would he have fared in 1968 if he had not sold this stock? In 1953, Sharp & Dohme and Merck & Company merged. At the time, 100 shares of Sharp & Dohme stock had a value of $4,500.00. Merck, as the surviving company, issued 2¼ shares of Merck stock for each share of Sharp & Dohme stock. Our investor thus owned 225 shares of Merck stock in 1953. In 1964, Merck stock was split 3 for 1, so that the investor now owned 675 shares of Merck stock. On April 23, 1968, a share of Merck stock sold for $88.50. The investor's shares thus had a value of $59,737.50.

Of course, if the investor had sold his stock on April 23, he would have had to pay a capital gains tax, which could not have exceeded 25 percent of the capital gain, however. The capital gain was $59,737.50 - $325.00 = $59,412.50. Twenty five percent of this is $14,853.13. The investor thus would have realized a profit after taxes of $59,412.50 − $14,853.13 = $44,559.37. In addition, of course, he received regular dividends each year. In 1968, the Merck dividend was $1.60 per share, so his dividends for the year were 675 x $1.60 = $1,080. The dividend earned in 1968 thus was 333 percent of the original investment. During the period 1953 to 1968, the value of a share of Merck stock increased approximately 13-fold.

I became affiliated with the Warner-Lambert Pharmaceutical Company in 1958. In the period 1958-1968, the value of a share of Warner-Lambert stock increased approximately 5-fold. At the Company's annual stockholder's meeting on April 16, 1968, Mr. Elmer Bobst, Honorary Board Chairman, stated that the annual sales of the Company had increased 24-fold since 1946 —from $29 million to $656 million. Profits increased 50-fold in this period. Warner-Lambert has become a highly diversified company, and the sales of ethical drugs accounted for only

24 percent of sales worldwide. However, Warner-Chilcott Laboratories, the Company's ethical marketing division in the United States, increased its sales 138 percent over the past 10 years. It is estimated that the ethical drug industry in this country will grow more than 50 percent over the next five years.

As I review these figures, I believe that they show that the rate of growth in the ethical drug industry is slower today than it was 20 years ago. But it still is a very healthy rate. My hunch is that stocks in this industry will continue to be valuable as growth stocks, although the rate of growth in the future will be slower than in the past.

◦§ §◦

And now we have reached the end. Thank you for reading this little book. As you must have realized by now, I believe that research in the ethical pharmaceutical industry is the most exciting and rewarding area in all of industry. I hope that some of my enthusiasm for the present and the past, as well as my optimism for the future, has rubbed off on you.

INDEX

Index